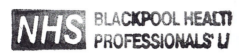 
FRCR Part 1
MCQs and Key Concepts

FRCR Part 1
MCQs and Key Concepts

William King MBBS BSc (Hons) MRCP
Specialist Registrar in Clinical Radiology
Southampton University Hospitals NHS Trust

AND

Amanda Williams MBBS MRCS
Specialist Registrar in Clinical Radiology
Portsmouth Hospitals NHS Trust

Edited for scientific content by

Catrin Abercrombie MSc CSci MIPEM
Medical Physicist
Portsmouth Hospitals NHS Trust

AND

Alistair Thomson BM MRCSEd
Specialist Registrar in Clinical Radiology
Portsmouth Hospitals NHS Trust

Radcliffe Publishing
Oxford • New York

Radcliffe Publishing Ltd
18 Marcham Road
Abingdon
Oxon OX14 1AA
United Kingdom

www.radcliffe-oxford.com
Electronic catalogue and worldwide online ordering facility.

British Library Cataloguing in Publication Data

A catalogue record for this book is available from the British Library.

ISBN-13: 978 184619 229 6

Typeset by Pindar New Zealand (Egan Reid), Auckland, New Zealand
Printed and bound by TJI Digital, Padstow, Cornwall, UK

Contents

Preface

The FRCR Part 1 examination is a challenging exam. The candidate needs to understand the key concepts behind the questions in order to succeed. The aim of our book is to provide a text which is a bridge between a pure MCQ based book and a physics textbook. Our book does not replace a physics textbook but we hope it will go a long way in providing enough understanding to pass the exam. We have written the questions to cover all areas examined by the FRCR Part 1 syllabus. Key concept notes and diagrams are provided to supplement the answers.

This book is written by two radiology registrars who have recently passed the FRCR Part 1. We are very appreciative of our editors who have supported us in producing what we believe is a high-quality concise revision aid.

William King and Amanda Williams
September 2007

List of abbreviations

α	alpha
A	atomic mass
ACoP	Approved Code of Practice
ARSAC	Administration of Radioactive Substances Advisory Committee
β	beta
Bq	Becquerel
CCD	charged couple device
CTDI	CT Dose Index
$CTDI_W$	weighted CT dose index
DLP	dose length product
DSA	digital subtraction angiography
EPD	electronic personal dosimeter
ESD	entrance surface dose
eV	electron volts
γ	gamma
Gy	gray
HSE	Health and Safety Executive
HU	Hounsfield unit
HVL	half-value layer
IR(ME)(A)R	Ionising Radiation (Medical Exposure) (Amendment) Regulations
IR(ME)R	Ionising Radiation (Medical Exposure) Regulations
IRR	Ionising Radiation Regulations
kV	kilovolts
kVp	peak tube voltage
LAC	linear attenuation coefficient
LET	linear energy transfer
LMP	last menstrual period
MBq	megabecquerel

MGD	mean glandular dose
Pb	lead
PET	positron emission tomography
PPE	personal protective equipment
PSP	photostimulable phosphor plate
QA	quality assurance
QC	quality control
RPA	Radiation Protection Advisor
RPS	Radiation Protection Supervisor
SNR	signal to noise ratio
SPECT	single photon emission computed tomography
Sv	sievert
$t_{1/2}$	half-life
TFT	thin film transistor
TLD	thermoluminescent dosimeter
Z	atomic number

CHAPTER 1

Basic physics

Q1.1 CONCERNING THE ATOM

A   All atoms contain protons and neutrons.

B   The atomic number is the sum of both neutrons and protons.

C   Electrons orbit around the nucleus in specific energy level regions called shells.

D   The innermost electrons orbiting in the K shell of the sodium atom are responsible for its chemical properties.

E   It is possible to remove electrons from orbiting shells and create ionised atoms.

Q1.2 CONCERNING PARTICLE INTERACTIONS

A A positron colliding with an electron will result in total annihilation of both particles.

B Gamma photons with 40 keV can remove K shell electrons from a tungsten atom.

C Protons with sufficient energy can be forced into a nucleus.

D During the process of electron capture it is typical for a beta particle to be emitted.

E The backward recoil of an electron during a Compton scattering event removes a greater proportion of the energy from the incident photon compared to a forward recoil event.

Q1.3 THE FOLLOWING STATEMENTS REGARDING X-RAY INTERACTION EVENTS ARE CORRECT

A An incident photon can collide with a bound electron without losing any energy.

B Photoelectric absorption is a characteristic radiation emitting process.

C Compton scattered photons can be scattered up to 180 degrees.

D The higher the initial energy of the photon during Compton scatter the higher its penetrance.

E During photoelectric absorption the incident photon gives up approximately 90% of its energy.

Q1.4 THE FOLLOWING ENTITIES HAVE MASS

A An alpha particle.

B A positron.

C   The resulting moiety after a positron interacts with an electron.

D   A gamma photon.

E   A high speed neutron from a cyclotron.

Q1.5 GAMMA PHOTONS

A   Are released from a rotating anode overcouch system when a high voltage current is passed across the tube.

B   Can be considered as both a particle and a wave.

C   If sufficiently energetic can remove electrons from their orbiting shell around a nucleus.

D   Can be emitted by an atom without changing its atomic mass or number.

E   Are more penetrative than alpha and beta radiation.

Q1.6 CONCERNING THE INTERACTION OF PHOTONS WITH MATTER

A   The predominant mode of interaction in air is Compton.

B   The predominant mode of interaction in soft tissue is photoelectric.

C   The predominant mode of interaction in contrast agent is Compton.

D   The mode of interaction in bone is both Compton and photoelectric.

E   The predominant mode of interaction in x-ray film is photoelectric.

Q1.7 THE FOLLOWING ARE TRUE OF ISOTOPES

A All isotopes of a given element have the same atomic mass.

B Isotopes of an element can have differing numbers of orbiting electrons.

C All isotopes have the same number of valence electrons.

D If the isotope has an unstable nucleus it is called a radioisotope.

E All isotopes of a given element have differing atomic numbers.

Q1.8 THE FOLLOWING STATEMENTS REGARDING NUCLEONS ARE TRUE

A Electron capture results in a reduction of the atomic number by one.

B Electron capture results in the emission of photons.

C Nuclides with a neutron deficit decay by converting a proton into a neutron.

D During beta negative decay a neutron is transformed into a proton.

E Mass and charge are conserved in proton to neutron conversion.

Q1.9 RADIOACTIVE DECAY

A Requires an unstable nucleus.

B Requires energy.

C Can be increased by superheating a radionuclide.

D Is guaranteed to occur in any radionuclide atom.

E Can be used to produce diagnostic images.

Q1.10 THE FOLLOWING STATEMENTS REGARDING RADIOACTIVITY ARE TRUE

A For a given quantity of radionuclide one can predict how long it will take for half of it to decay.

B One million decays per second equals one megabecquerel (1 MBq).

C The radioactivity of a radionuclide decreases by equal percentages in equal intervals of time.

D The radioactivity of a sample will eventually reach zero.

E After 10 half-lives the radioactivity of a sample will be a tenth of its original activity.

Q1.11 THE FOLLOWING ARE MODES OF INTERACTION BETWEEN X-RAYS AND GAMMA RAYS WITH MATTER

A Translocation.

B Transmission.

C Convection.

D Absorption.

E Scatter.

Q1.12 THE FOLLOWING ARE TRUE OF ATTENUATION

A Attenuation = Transmission – Scatter.

B Attenuation = Absorption + Scatter.

C Attenuation = Transmission multiplied by the linear attenuation coefficient.

D Attenuation = Incident beam – Attenuated beam.

E Attenuation = Tissue weighting factor.

Q1.13 THE FOLLOWING STATEMENTS ARE TRUE OF THE LINEAR ATTENUATION COEFFICIENT AND ITS CALCULATION

A The linear attenuation coefficient (LAC) is the fractional reduction in intensity of a monoenergetic beam of x-ray or gamma radiation per unit thickness of attenuating material.

B The LAC is constant for the attenuating material whether in solid or liquid state.

C The LAC is dependent on density.

D The LAC is measured in kV.

E Can only be approximated for a beam of x-rays as the beam is not perfectly monoenergetic.

Q1.14 THE FOLLOWING ARE TRUE OF THE 'HALF VALUE LAYER' (HVL)

A It is the thickness of a certain material that reduces the intensity of a monoenergetic beam of x-rays or gamma radiation by half.

B The HVL is inversely proportional to the linear attenuation coefficient.

C The HVL decreases if the density of the attenuating material decreases.

D   The HVL decreases with a lower mean photon energy of the beam.

E   The HVL decreases with decreased atomic number of the attenuating material.

Q1.15 THE FOLLOWING ARE TRUE OF ELECTROMAGNETIC RADIATION

A   It travels in straight lines unless attenuated.

B   The intensity of radiation emitted from a point source will reduce in inverse proportion to the square of the distance from that point source.

C   The frequency of electromagnetic radiation is inversely proportional to its wavelength.

D   If the intensity of radiation 1 m from a point source is 50% the intensity will be reduced to 25% at 2 m.

E   The inverse square law will predict the reduction in intensity of a beam of radiation from a point source passing through lead.

Q1.16 IF THE HALF-LIFE OF A SOURCE OF 20 MBQ IS ONE HOUR

A   At two hours its activity will be 10 MBq.

B   At four hours its activity will be 1.25 MBq.

C   At 25 hours the source will cease to be radioactive.

D   Heating the source will reduce the half-life.

E   A constant number of the radionuclide's atoms will decay at any one time.

Q1.17 THE FOLLOWING DECAY PROCESSES DO NOT RESULT IN A CHANGE OF ATOMIC NUMBER (Z)

A β^- decay.

B Isomeric transition.

C β^+ decay.

D Internal conversion.

E K shell capture.

Q1.18 THE FOLLOWING ARE TRUE OF K SHELL ABSORPTION EDGES

A Incident photons of lower energy can be attenuated less than those of higher energies.

B The K-edge binding energy is always greater than the L-edge binding energy for a given element.

C Filtering material will be relatively transparent to its own K-edge characteristic radiation.

D The phenomenon is of no use in diagnostic imaging.

E L and M-edge characteristic radiation from tungsten is useful in image formation.

Q1.19 THE FOLLOWING ARE TRUE OF PHOTOELECTRIC ABSORPTION

A It is the predominant mode of absorption by iodine based contrast agents.

B All the energy of the incident photon is transferred to the ejected electron.

C   The incident photon is greatly reduced in energy during the interaction process.

D   Having ejected an electron the atom becomes ionised.

E   Results in the emission of Bremsstrahlung radiation.

Q1.20 CONCERNING COMPTON SCATTER

A   It is also known as modified scatter.

B   Can result in total absorption of the incident photon.

C   Can occur with any bound electron.

D   Is dependent on the atomic number of the attenuating material.

E   Is dependent on the density of the attenuating material.

Q1.21 THE FOLLOWING ARE FORMS OF ELECTROMAGNETIC RADIATION

A   Gamma radiation.

B   Radio waves.

C   Blue light.

D   Alpha radiation.

E   X-rays.

Q1.22 THE FOLLOWING ARE TRUE OF PHOTONS

A   They can be considered as both a wave and a particle.

B   They all have the same frequency.

C   Their velocity can be slowed by passing through a gas.

D   If travelling through a vacuum their speed will be constant.

E   If supercooled they have mass.

Q1.23 THE BINDING ENERGY OF AN ORBITING ELECTRON

A   For a given atom is greater for a K shell electron than an M shell electron.

B   Can be overcome if bombarded with an electron of greater energy.

C   Is normally measured in joules.

D   Is the same as the kinetic energy of the orbiting electron.

E   Increases the further an electron orbits from the nucleus.

Q1.24 THE TOTAL NUMBER OF NUCLEONS IN A NUCLEUS IS ALWAYS EQUAL TO

A   The atomic number.

B   The number of orbiting electrons.

C   The atomic mass.

D   Its position on the periodic table.

E   The sum of protons and electrons.

Q1.25 PROTONS

A   Are negatively charged.

B   Have a relative mass.

C   For a given atom are matched in number by orbiting electrons.

D   For some atoms can be the only component of the nucleus.

E   Can be described as a nucleon.

Q1.26 THE FOLLOWING ENTITIES ARE COMPONENTS FOUND IN THE NUCLEUS

A   Electrons.

B   Positrons.

C   Protons.

D   Photons.

E   Neutrons.

Q1.27 THE FOLLOWING ARE TRUE OF ELECTRON SHELLS

A   These are orbits around a nucleus that contain electrons.

B   The K shell can contain four electrons.

C   The L shell can contain eight electrons.

D   The maximum capacity of the M shell is 18 electrons.

E   The outermost shell containing electrons is called the valence shell.

Q1.28 REGARDING THE HALF-LIFE OF A GIVEN QUANTITY OF A PARTICULAR RADIONUCLIDE

A It is constant.

B It is the time for half of the radionuclide at a given time to decay into its daughter product.

C If the half-life is short the radioactivity will be relatively low.

D It can be reduced by superheating the radionuclide.

E It can be reduced by chemically bonding the radionuclide to a protein.

Q1.29 RADIOACTIVE DECAY

A Of an individual radionuclide atom can be predicted.

B Can be reduced by supercooling.

C Is a statistically predictable process.

D The half-life is increased if the radionuclide nucleus is more unstable.

E Is an exponentially decreasing process.

Q1.30 CONCERNING SECONDARY ELECTRONS

A They are produced by photoelectric absorption.

B They are produced by Compton scattering events.

C They create ion pairs.

D The range of secondary electrons is directly proportional to the density of the material they are passing through.

E A typical track of a secondary electron is straight when passing through matter.

TVO 5690

Answers

A1.1 CONCERNING THE ATOM

A False – Hydrogen only has one proton and one electron.

B False.

C True.

D False – It is the electrons in the outermost shell or 'valence' shell that are predominantly responsible for the chemical properties.

E True – This is called ionisation.

A1.2 CONCERNING PARTICLE INTERACTIONS

A True – All their mass is converted into energy in the form of two gamma rays which travel in opposite directions at 180 degrees to each other.

B False – The K shell binding energy of tungsten is 70 keV and needs to be exceeded to remove an electron from this shell.

C True – This occurs within a cyclotron.

D False – During electron capture only gamma photons are emitted.

E False – No electron is recoiled backwards during a Compton scattering event.

A1.3 THE FOLLOWING STATEMENTS REGARDING X-RAY INTERACTION EVENTS ARE CORRECT

A True – This is called elastic, unmodified or coherent scatter.

B True.

C True.

D True.

E False – Photoelectric absorption is total absorption. The incident photon no longer exists.

KEY CONCEPT

CONSTITUENTS OF THE ATOM

The atom of an element contains a very small nucleus surrounded by orbiting electrons. The electrons orbit within 'shells' which have distinct energy levels. The nucleus has a positive charge and the electrons have a negative charge. Thus the electrons are held in orbit. The closer the shell is to the nucleus the more tightly its orbiting electrons are held. The nucleus contains protons and neutrons which are collectively described as nucleons.

Protons:	Have a relative charge of +1 and a relative mass of 1.
Neutrons:	Have a charge of 0 and a relative mass of 1.
Electrons:	Have a charge of −1 and a relative mass of 1/1840.
Atomic number (Z):	Is the number of protons in the nucleus and thus the number of orbiting electrons. It defines the name of the element.
Atomic mass (A):	Is the mass of the nucleus and is the sum of the protons and neutrons.
Binding energy:	Is the energy required to completely remove an electron from its shell and parent atom. It is expressed as electron volts or eV. The closer the orbiting electron to the nucleus the greater the binding energy.
Ionisation:	Is defined as the complete removal of an electron from its parent atom. The electron will have a charge of −1 and the parent atom +1. The parent is described as being 'ionised'.
Isotopes:	Atoms with the same atomic number but differing mass numbers.

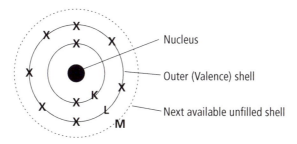

FIGURE 1.1 A fluorine atom and its surrounding shells

KEY CONCEPT

IONISING RADIATION AND ITS FORMS

Ionising radiation describes a group of entities that have sufficient energy to ionise (remove) electrons from atoms they interact with. In living organisms this can lead to cellular damage.

Alpha particles (α): Are high speed helium atoms (A=4, Z=2) with a charge of +2. They are highly ionising but only travel short distances through material before being stopped.

Beta particles (β⁻): Are high speed electrons emitted by unstable nuclei and have a charge of −1. They have a relative atomic mass of 1/1840.

Positrons (β⁺): Are high speed positive electrons emitted by unstable nuclei and have a charge of +1. They have a relative atomic mass of 1/1840.

X-rays and gamma rays (γ): Are distinct 'packets' of electromagnetic radiation called photons. Electromagnetic radiation does not have mass or charge but has energy. They can be thought of as particles or waves which is the basis of the 'wave-particle' theory of electromagnetic radiation.

A1.4 THE FOLLOWING ENTITIES HAVE MASS

A   True.

B   True.

C   False.

D   False.

E   True.

A1.5 GAMMA PHOTONS

A   False – This is the principle behind x-ray production.

B   True – This is the 'wave-particle' theory of gamma radiation.

C   True – This is the basis of photoelectric absorption.

D   True – An example of this is technetium-99m.

E   True.

> **KEY CONCEPT**
>
> ## THE DIFFERENCE BETWEEN GAMMA AND X-RAYS
>
> Even though gamma and x-ray photons are identical entities they are differentiated from each other by their origin. Gamma rays are produced by spontaneous nuclear stabilising events and x-rays are produced by bombarding anodes with high speed electrons.

A1.6 CONCERNING THE INTERACTION OF PHOTONS WITH MATTER

A True.

B False – The Compton effect predominates.

C False – Contrast agents have a high atomic number and therefore the photoelectric effect predominates.

D True – Bone has differing regions of atomic number (i.e. marrow vs. cortex), therefore a mixture of absorption occurs.

E True.

A1.7 THE FOLLOWING ARE TRUE OF ISOTOPES

A False.

B False – The number of electrons is dependent on the quantity of protons.

C True.

D True.

E False.

A1.8 THE FOLLOWING STATEMENTS REGARDING NUCLEONS ARE TRUE

A True.

B True.

C True.

D True – An electron is also emitted.

E True.

KEY CONCEPT

NUCLEAR STABILISATION EVENTS

Electron capture (neutron deficit): A nucleus can be unstable because it contains too few neutrons. One of the protons may capture one of the atom's innermost orbiting electrons and convert into a neutron. The atomic number (Z) will reduce by one but the atomic mass (A) will remain the same. The captured electron leaves a vacancy within the innermost shell. This is filled with an outer shell electron dropping into its place. A photon of energy is released as a result. The photon's energy will be the difference between the energy levels of these two shells.

β⁻ decay (neutron excess): A nucleus can be unstable because it has too many neutrons. A neutron can change into a proton and an electron. The electron is ejected from the nucleus at high speed and so is by definition a beta particle. The atomic mass (A) remains the same; however, the atomic number (Z) increases by one.

β⁺ decay (neutron deficit): A nucleus can be unstable because it has too few neutrons. A proton can change into a neutron and a positive electron (positron) rendering the nucleus more stable. The atomic number (Z) decreases by one; the atomic mass (A) remains the same.

Isomeric transition: This is when a nucleus is still in an excited state after a decay event. This is described as a 'metastable' state. It will eventually stabilise to its ground state with the emission of a gamma photon. An example of this is technetium-99m which stabilises to technetium-99 with the emission of a 140 keV gamma photon.

A1.9 RADIOACTIVE DECAY

A True.

B False – If a nucleus is unstable it will decay spontaneously.

C False – Physical and chemical conditions will not affect radioactivity.

D False – Radioactive decay is a random unpredictable event.

E True – This is the principle of nuclear imaging.

A1.10 THE FOLLOWING STATEMENTS REGARDING RADIOACTIVITY ARE TRUE

A   True – This is known as the half-life.

B   True – The unit Becquerel (1 Bq) defines the number of decays per second.

C   True – This is exponential decay.

D   False – Radioactivity decay is exponential so it will never reach zero.

E   False – It will be 1/1024.

A1.11 THE FOLLOWING ARE MODES OF INTERACTION BETWEEN X-RAYS AND GAMMA RAYS WITH MATTER

A   False – This process is involved in DNA replication.

B   True – The photons pass directly through with no loss of energy or altered trajectory.

C   False – This is a mode of heat transmission.

D   True.

E   True.

A1.12 THE FOLLOWING ARE TRUE OF ATTENUATION

A   False.

B   True.

C   False.

D   True.

E   False – The tissue weighting factor represents how susceptible a certain tissue is to radiation damage.

KEY CONCEPT

ABSORPTION, SCATTER, TRANSMISSION AND ATTENUATION

Absorption: The photon completely transfers all its energy to the matter.

Partial absorption: The photon transfers some of its energy to the matter.

Scatter: The photon's course is altered due to an interaction with the atoms of the matter. Scattered photons may also lose some energy to the matter.

Transmission: The photon is unattenuated by and passes directly through the matter.

Attenuation: Is the total number of photons that have been removed from the primary beam after passing through the attenuating material. They can be attenuated either by scatter or absorption.

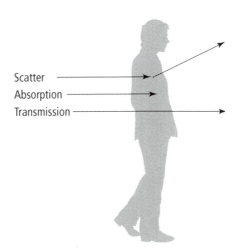

Scatter

Absorption

Transmission

FIGURE 1.2 Three possible modes of interaction between x-rays and gamma rays with matter

A1.13 THE FOLLOWING STATEMENTS ARE TRUE OF THE LINEAR ATTENUATION COEFFICIENT AND ITS CALCULATION

A True.

B False – It is dependent on the density of the material.

C True.

D False.

E True.

A1.14 THE FOLLOWING ARE TRUE OF THE 'HALF VALUE LAYER' (HVL)

A True.

B True – HVL = 0.69/LAC.

C False – It will increase.

D True – The photons are less energetic and are attenuated more easily, therefore the HVL will decrease.

E False – If the atomic number of the attenuating material is decreased the HVL will increase.

A1.15 THE FOLLOWING ARE TRUE OF ELECTROMAGNETIC RADIATION

A True.

B True – This is the inverse square law.

C True.

D False – It will be 12.5% using the inverse square law.

E False – Absorption and scatter will further remove photons from the beam thus the intensity of the beam will be far less than that calculated using the inverse square law.

KEY CONCEPT

THE INVERSE SQUARE LAW

States that the intensity of radiation emitted from a point source will reduce in inverse proportion to the square of the distance from that point source.

A useful way to think about it is that for every doubling of distance from a point source its intensity will decrease by a quarter each time.

So $1/4 \Rightarrow 1/16 \Rightarrow 1/64$.

A1.16 IF THE HALF-LIFE OF A SOURCE OF 20 MBQ IS ONE HOUR

A False – It will be 5 MBq as two half-lives have passed at two hours.

B True – Four half-lives will have passed.

C False – Radioactivity will never fall to zero as it follows exponential decay.

D False – Radioactivity is independent of physical and chemical conditions.

E False – As the radionuclide decays less of the original atoms will be present to decay.

A1.17 THE FOLLOWING DECAY PROCESSES DO NOT RESULT IN A CHANGE OF ATOMIC NUMBER (Z)

A False – The atomic number increases by one as a neutron is converted into a proton.

B True.

C False – In a nucleus with a neutron deficit, a proton will convert into a neutron and emit a β^+ particle.

D True – A gamma photon emitted by a nucleus can be photoelectrically absorbed by its K shell orbiting electrons, thus emitting characteristic radiation.

E False – K shell capture is electron capture. A nucleus with a deficit of neutrons relative to protons can convert a nuclear proton into a neutron by capturing a K shell electron.

A1.18 THE FOLLOWING ARE TRUE OF K SHELL ABSORPTION EDGES

A True – This phenomenon explains the K-edge jump on absorption spectrum graphs.

B True – The K shell electrons have a greater binding energy.

C True.

D False – K-edge filters are used to remove low energy radiation which contributes to patient dose.

E False – For tungsten L-edge radiation is <12 keV and M-edge radiation is <2 KeV and therefore it is useless in image formation.

A1.19 THE FOLLOWING ARE TRUE OF PHOTOELECTRIC ABSORPTION

A   True.

B   False – Some of the energy is required to overcome the binding energy.

C   False – It disappears.

D   True – This may result in tissue damage.

E   False – It results in the production of characteristic radiation.

A1.20 CONCERNING COMPTON SCATTER

A   True.

B   False – Modified scatter is a partial absorption process.

C   False – It only occurs with free or loosely bound electrons

D   False – It is dependent on density and not atomic number.

E   True.

KEY CONCEPT

PHOTOELECTRIC ABSORPTION VS. COMPTON SCATTER

Photoelectric absorption: Inner orbital electrons are ejected by an incident photon with sufficient energy. Electrons from outer shells then drop into the ejected inner electron's vacant position. This results in the emission of a photon of characteristic radiation.

- Involves inner bound orbital atomic electrons.
- Results in complete photon absorption.
- Results in atomic ionisation.
- Results in the emission of characteristic radiation.
- Is dependent on atomic number Z (i.e. the number of orbiting bound electrons).

Compton scatter: A photon interacts with a free electron which recoils taking away some of the energy as kinetic energy.

- Involves free electrons.
- Only results in partial absorption of the incident photons energy.
- Is **dependent** on the physical density of the attenuating material and is **independent** of the atomic number of the material.

A1.21 THE FOLLOWING ARE FORMS OF ELECTROMAGNETIC RADIATION

A True.

B True.

C True.

D False – An alpha particle is a helium atom.

E True.

A1.22 THE FOLLOWING ARE TRUE OF PHOTONS

A True.

B False – Photons have differing frequencies which define the type of radiation.

C True – Electromagnetic radiation is slowed when passing through different substances.

D True.

E False – Electromagnetic radiation has no mass.

A1.23 THE BINDING ENERGY OF AN ORBITING ELECTRON

A True.

B True – This is how characteristic radiation is produced.

C False – It is usually measured in electron volts.

D False.

E False – The further the orbiting electron from the positive nuclear force the less tightly it is held.

A1.24 THE TOTAL NUMBER OF NUCLEONS IN A NUCLEUS IS ALWAYS EQUAL TO

A False.

B False.

C True.

D False – The periodic table is a chart of all known elements and laid out by atomic number.

E False.

A1.25 PROTONS

A False.

B True.

C True.

D True – The hydrogen atom contains only one lone proton in its nucleus.

E True.

A1.26 THE FOLLOWING ENTITIES ARE COMPONENTS FOUND IN THE NUCLEUS

A False.

B False.

C True.

D False.

E True.

A1.27 THE FOLLOWING ARE TRUE OF ELECTRON SHELLS

A True.

B False – Its maximum holding capacity is two electrons.

C True.

D True.

E True – This is responsible for the chemical properties of the atom.

A1.28 REGARDING THE HALF-LIFE OF A GIVEN QUANTITY OF A PARTICULAR RADIONUCLIDE

A True.

B True.

C False – The radionuclide will be highly radioactive if it has a short half-life.

D False – Radioactivity is not affected by chemical or physical conditions.

E False – As above.

A1.29 RADIOACTIVE DECAY

A False – Radioactive decay is a random process.

B False – Radioactivity is not affected by any chemical or physical conditions.

C True.

D False – The more unstable a nucleus is the more likely it is to decay and therefore the half-life will be shorter.

E True.

A1.30 CONCERNING SECONDARY ELECTRONS

A True – Electrons are ejected during photoelectric absorption.

B True – The incident photons scatter free electrons.

C True – As they strike valence electrons they displace them and ionise the atom creating ion pairs.

D False – It is inversely proportional.

E False – It will follow a random course due to numerous interactions with other electrons.

CHAPTER 2

Radiation hazards and dosimetry

Q2.1 RADIOBIOLOGICAL DAMAGE TO TISSUE

A Is caused by an ionisation event directly rupturing a covalent bond.

B Is induced by the production of free radicals causing molecular damage.

C Occurs by the absorption of energy from ionising radiation damaging DNA.

D Is dependent on the radiosensitivity of the tissue.

E Depends on the linear energy transfer (LET).

Q2.2 REGARDING THE BIOLOGICAL EFFECTS OF RADIATION

A   A high radiation absorbed dose of 1 Gy is used in radiotherapy to destroy malignant cells.

B   Damage to biological tissue occurs by the deposition of large amounts of energy.

C   Radiation can damage cell membranes causing changes in permeability and motility.

D   Electron binding energy needs to be exceeded to cause ionisation.

E   Tissues with a static cell population are more sensitive to radiation damage.

Q2.3 CONCERNING THE BIOLOGICAL RISKS OF RADIATION

A   DNA is the only structure damaged by radiation.

B   X-rays and gamma rays produce the most biological damage from external exposure.

C   Alpha particles cause the least biological damage from internal exposure following ingestion.

D   Alpha particles produce the most biological damage from external exposure as they are unable to penetrate the skin.

E   Beta particles can penetrate the skin and cause damage.

Q2.4 REGARDING RISKS OF RADIATION

A   Radiation damage to cells is less severe if the dose is delivered in fractions.

B   Replicating cells are less susceptible to cell damage than static cell populations due to their high turnover.

C   Radiation weighting factors are used to account for the greater effective-
    ness of some radiation in producing biological damage.

D   Cells are able to repair almost all radiation damage at low dose rates.

E   High LET radiation such as alpha particles create ionisation events close
    together and so can break both strands of DNA.

Q2.5 CONCERNING THE RISKS OF RADIATION

A   The average effective dose received per annum by an individual in the
    UK is 2.7 Sv.

B   Each individual receives on average an effective dose of 2.3 Sv per
    annum from natural sources.

C   The average effective dose received per annum by an individual in the
    UK is 2.7 mSv.

D   The effective dose of a PA CXR is 0.2 mSv.

E   The effective dose of a CT of the abdomen is 5 mSv.

Q2.6 THE FOLLOWING ARE DETERMINISTIC EFFECTS OF IONISING RADIATION

A   Erythema.

B   Leukaemia.

C   Cataracts.

D   Prodromal syndrome.

E   Bowel malignancy.

Q2.7 CONCERNING DETERMINISTIC EFFECTS IN DIGITAL SUBTRACTION ANGIOGRAPHY

A The threshold dose for transient erythema of the skin is 4 Gy.

B Permanent epilation occurs above a threshold dose of 6 Gy.

C Dermal necrosis occurs above a threshold dose of 14 Gy.

D The threshold dose for dry desquamation of the skin is 18 Gy.

E The time of onset of effects from radiation exposure may be prolonged.

Q2.8 DETERMINISTIC EFFECTS

A Include cataracts.

B Include hereditary effects.

C The severity of the deterministic effect increases with increasing dose of radiation.

D The probability of the effect increases with increasing dose.

E Only occur above a dose threshold.

Q2.9 DURING INTERVENTIONAL RADIOLOGICAL PROCEDURES THE FOLLOWING DETERMINISTIC EFFECTS CAN OCCUR

A Permanent sterility.

B Epilation.

C Erythema.

D Breast cancer.

E Skin ulceration.

Q2.10 THE FOLLOWING ARE STOCHASTIC EFFECTS OF RADIATION

A Breast cancer.

B Infertility.

C Skin ulceration.

D Temporary loss of haemopoiesis.

E Transient vomiting and diarrhoea.

Q2.11 STOCHASTIC EFFECTS

A Include epilation.

B Include breast cancer.

C The severity of the effect increases with increasing dose of radiation.

D The probability of the effect increases with increasing dose.

E Only occur above a dose threshold.

Q2.12 THE FOLLOWING RISK FACTORS ARE TRUE

A   The risk (number of individuals per 100 exposed to 1 Sv) of developing a fatal cancer is 5.

B   The risk (number of individuals per 100 exposed to 1 Sv) of developing a non-fatal cancer is 1.

C   The risk (number of individuals per 100 exposed to 1 Sv) of genetic effects is 1.3.

D   The risk of developing a fatal cancer from a CT head is 1 in 10 000.

E   The risk of developing a fatal cancer from a CT abdomen is 1 in 2000.

Q2.13 THE PRINCIPLES OF RADIATION PROTECTION STATE THAT

A   A decrease in distance from the source of radiation reduces the dose.

B   If the source of radiation is a point source, the dose reduction with distance obeys the inverse square law.

C   The shorter the exposure time, the lower the dose.

D   The thicker or denser the material, the better the shielding.

E   The shielding performance of most x-ray room walls, doors and windows should be constructed from material with a 2.5 cm Pb equivalence.

Q2.14 ESSENTIAL PROTECTIVE EQUIPMENT USED IN AN ANGIOGRAPHY SUITE INCLUDES

A   Lead aprons.

B   Thyroid shields.

C Finger dose monitors.

D Lead glasses.

E Protective screens.

Q2.15 CONCERNING RADIATION PROTECTION IN A CT SCANNING ROOM

A Any individual in the room during scanning must wear an apron of 0.25 mm Pb equivalent.

B The use of a thyroid collar has little effect on radiation protection.

C Extremity monitors can be used to measure dose to fingers close to the scan plane.

D The use of the lowest exposure factors reduces the dose received by the patient and the operator.

E Lead glasses are advocated when close to the scan plane.

Q2.16 EXPOSURE CAN BE RESTRICTED BY

A The use of lead plasterboard incorporated into the room design.

B The use of lead glasses when performing interventional studies.

C The use of lead aprons to reduce exposure to the primary beam.

D A regular quality assurance programme of equipment.

E The use of thyroid shields.

Q2.17 REGARDING RADIATION SAFETY IN RADIONUCLIDE IMAGING

A Internal radiation hazards arise from radioactive substances inside the body.

B The dose received from an external radiation hazard may be reduced by increasing the distance from the source.

C Radiation dose = Dose rate × Time.

D Time, distance and shielding can be used to limit the radiation dose received from external radiation.

E An external radiation hazard arises from sources of radiation outside the body.

Q2.18 THE FOLLOWING REDUCE THE RADIATION DOSE TO THE OPERATOR WHEN ADMINISTERING A RADIOPHARMACEUTICAL

A Using a syringe shield.

B Holding the syringe so that the activity is as far away as possible.

C Wearing gloves.

D Completing the procedure as fast as possible.

E Monitoring yourself after the procedure to check for contamination.

Q2.19 THE FOLLOWING PERSONAL PROTECTIVE EQUIPMENT (PPE) PROTECTS STAFF FROM THE UNATTENUATED PRIMARY RADIATION

A Lead gloves.

B Lead glasses.

C   Lead aprons.

D   Thyroid shields.

E   Lead shields.

Q2.20 CONCERNING RADIATION PROTECTION

A   During a fluoroscopic procedure a pulsed operation reduces the time of exposure to the primary beam.

B   A lead apron should have a lead equivalence of 0.25 mm for use of x-rays up to 150 kV.

C   The size of the radiation beam has no effect on the radiation dose received.

D   An overcouch system exposes the upper body to more scattered radiation than an undercouch system.

E   The radiation dose received by the operator will be less using an overcouch fluoroscopy configuration compared to an undercouch.

Q2.21 THE FOLLOWING FACTORS INFLUENCE THE ENTRANCE SURFACE DOSE

A   Image receptor dose.

B   Patient factors.

C   Film to focus distance.

D   Radiation quality.

E   Absorption of the beam after the patient.

Q2.22 REGARDING GENERAL RADIATION PROTECTION PRINCIPLES

A Control shields provide protection from the scattered radiation.

B The tube incorporates copper shielding to attenuate the radiation travelling in any direction other than the primary beam.

C The leakage radiation at 1 m from the focus must not total more than 10 mSv.

D X-ray rooms may have barium plaster on the walls to increase their shielding properties.

E The aim of radiation protection is to reduce deterministic effects only.

Q2.23 GENERAL RADIATION PROTECTION

A Thermoluminescent personal dosimeters (TLD) should be worn under lead aprons.

B Lead aprons protect individuals from the primary beam and radiation attenuated or scattered by the patient.

C Thyroid shields are only effective in very high dose procedures.

D Lead aprons are normally 2.5 mm of lead in thickness.

E When palpating a patient in the primary beam a lead glove of at least 0.25 mm Pb equivalent should be worn.

Q2.24 RADIATION PROTECTION OF STAFF AND MEMBERS OF THE PUBLIC

A X-ray rooms are permanently controlled areas.

B At the entrance to the x-ray room there is a warning sign to indicate a controlled area.

C   A carer is able to comfort a child but must wear protective clothing and be positioned outside of the primary beam.

D   Members of the public can receive up to 1 mSv per week.

E   X-ray protection to staff must be provided against the primary beam, leakage radiation and scattered radiation.

Q2.25 ABSORBED DOSE

A   Is measured in sieverts (Sv).

B   Is measured in gray (Gy).

C   Is the amount of energy imparted per unit mass to a medium by the incident ray.

D   Takes into account the difference in biological effects of different types of radiation.

E   Depends on the cumulated activity in the source organ and the fraction of energy absorbed in the target organ.

Q2.26 EQUIVALENT DOSE

A   Is the product of the effective dose multiplied by a tissue weighting factor.

B   Is measured in joules per kilogram.

C   Is measured in sieverts (Sv).

D   Is used to compare doses from different radiological techniques applied to a particular organ.

E   Is the product of the absorbed dose multiplied by a radiation weighting factor.

Q2.27 EFFECTIVE DOSE

A Is measured in gray (Gy).

B Is the product of the absorbed dose multiplied by a radiation weighting factor.

C Accounts for the difference in sensitivity of the tissue to radiation.

D Is always the same as the dose area product.

E Of a chest x-ray is 0.2 mSv.

Q2.28 THE TYPICAL EFFECTIVE DOSE FOR THE FOLLOWING PROCEDURES ARE

A CXR = 0.02 mSv.

B CT head = 2 mSv.

C Barium enema = 7 mSv.

D CT abdomen = 5 mSv.

E IVU = 2.5mSv.

Answers

A2.1 RADIOBIOLOGICAL DAMAGE TO TISSUE

A True – A direct effect of radiation.

B True – An indirect effect of radiation.

C True – A direct effect of radiation.

D True – Cells are radiosensitive and more susceptible to damage if they are mitotically active.

E True.

A2.2 REGARDING THE BIOLOGICAL EFFECTS OF RADIATION

A True.

B False.

C True.

D True.

E False – Tissues with a high cellular turnover tend to be more sensitive to radiation damage.

A2.3 CONCERNING THE BIOLOGICAL RISKS OF RADIATION

A False – Other cellular components can be damaged.

B False – Neutrons cause the most damage from external exposure.

C False – Alpha particles cause the most damage from internal exposure.

D False.

E True.

A2.4 REGARDING RISKS OF RADIATION

A True.

B False – The effects are more severe in cells with a high turnover.

C True.

D True.

E True.

A2.5 CONCERNING THE RISKS OF RADIATION

A False – The average effective dose is 2.7 mSv.

B False – Each individual receives on average 2.3 mSv per annum.

C True.

D False – The effective dose is 0.02 mSv.

E False – The effective dose is 10 mSv.

A2.6 THE FOLLOWING ARE DETERMINISTIC EFFECTS OF IONISING RADIATION

A True.

B False.

C True.

D True.

E False.

RELATIVE TISSUE RADIOSENSITIVITY

Radiosensitive tissues	Radio-resistant tissues
Bone marrow	Liver
Gut epithelium	Kidney
Germinal cells of the ovary and testis	Brain
	Connective tissue
Skin	Bone
Foetal tissues	Muscle
Many tumours	

KEY CONCEPT

LINEAR ENERGY TRANSFER

- Linear energy transfer (LET) is the deposition of energy along the track of a photon or particle.
- Low LET radiation includes x-rays, gamma rays and beta particles which are sparsely ionising.
- High LET radiation includes alpha particles and neutrons which are densely ionising.
- LET is useful to assess the biological consequences of different types of radiation.

A2.7 CONCERNING DETERMINISTIC EFFECTS IN DIGITAL SUBTRACTION ANGIOGRAPHY

A False.

B False.

C False.

D False.

E True.

A2.8 DETERMINISTIC EFFECTS

A True.

B False – This is a stochastic effect.

C True.

D False – This is true of stochastic effects.

E True.

A2.9 DURING INTERVENTIONAL RADIOLOGICAL PROCEDURES THE FOLLOWING DETERMINISTIC EFFECTS CAN OCCUR

A False – Theoretically this is possible but is unlikely with the amount received for diagnostic procedures.

B True.

C True.

D False – This is a stochastic effect.

E True.

KEY CONCEPT

THRESHOLD DOSES OF SKIN DAMAGE

	Threshold dose (Gy)	Time of onset
Transient erythema	2	2–24 hours
Main erythema reaction	6	10 days
Permanent epilation	7	3 weeks
Dry desquamation	14	4 weeks
Dermal necrosis	18	52 weeks

A2.10 THE FOLLOWING ARE STOCHASTIC EFFECTS OF RADIATION

A True.

B False.

C False.

D False.

E False.

A2.11 STOCHASTIC EFFECTS

A False – This is a deterministic effect.

B True.

C False – This is true of deterministic effects.

D True.

E False – This is true of deterministic effects.

A2.12 THE FOLLOWING RISK FACTORS ARE TRUE

A True.

B True.

C True.

D True.

E True.

KEY CONCEPT

STOCHASTIC AND DETERMINISTIC EFFECTS

- **Stochastic** (statistical) effects are due to genetic mutations resulting in an increased probability of neoplasia. The probability of incidence is proportional to radiation dose.
- **Deterministic** (threshold) effects are due to direct tissue damage by radiation once a certain dose threshold is reached. Once the threshold is exceeded the severity of the effect increases with increasing dose. Recovery can occur.

Deterministic effects	Threshold dose (Gy)
Prodromal syndrome	0.5
Erythema	2.0
Hair loss	3.0
Cataracts	2–5
Ovulation suppression	1.5–5
Temporary loss of sperm	0.3–2

A2.13 THE PRINCIPLES OF RADIATION PROTECTION STATE THAT

A False – An increase in distance from the source reduces the dose.

B True.

C True.

D True.

E False – Materials should have approximately 2–2.5 mm Pb equivalence. However, purpose built rooms take into account workload, occupancy of the surrounding area and technique employed.

A2.14 ESSENTIAL PROTECTIVE EQUIPMENT USED IN AN ANGIOGRAPHY SUITE INCLUDES

A True – Staff in angiography rooms have the potential to receive extremely high doses.

B True.

C True.

D True.

E True.

A2.15 CONCERNING RADIATION PROTECTION IN A CT SCANNING ROOM

A False – An apron of 0.35 mm Pb is required.

B False – A thyroid collar should be worn.

C True.

D True.

E True.

A2.16 EXPOSURE CAN BE RESTRICTED BY

A True – 1 mm lead = 12 mm barium plaster = 120 mm concrete.

B True.

C False – Lead aprons protect you from scattered radiation only.

D True – This ensures the equipment is working properly.

E True.

A2.17 REGARDING RADIATION SAFETY IN RADIONUCLIDE IMAGING

A True.

B True.

C True.

D True.

E True.

A2.18 THE FOLLOWING REDUCE THE RADIATION DOSE TO THE OPERATOR WHEN ADMINISTERING A RADIOPHARMACEUTICAL

A True – Shielding.

B True – Distance.

C False – Gloves are used predominantly to reduce contamination.

D True – Time.

E True.

A2.19 THE FOLLOWING PERSONAL PROTECTIVE EQUIPMENT (PPE) PROTECTS STAFF FROM THE UNATTENUATED PRIMARY RADIATION

A False.

B False.

C False.

D False.

E False.

KEY CONCEPT

PRINCIPLES OF RADIATION PROTECTION

The three principles of radiation protection are **time**, **distance** and **shielding**.

- The shorter the exposure time, the lower the dose received.
- The intensity of a beam of electromagnetic radiation from a point source reduces with the square of the distance from the source. The radiation becomes spread out and therefore the intensity is reduced – this is the inverse square law.
- The thicker or denser the material, the better the shielding. This is described in terms of its lead equivalence. The units are millimetres of lead (mm Pb) and should state at what energy level this applies.

A2.20 CONCERNING RADIATION PROTECTION

A True.

B False – A lead apron should have a lead equivalence of 0.35 mm for x-rays up to 150 kV and 0.25 mm lead equivalence up to 100 kV.

C False – The size of the radiation beam should be kept as small as possible to limit the radiation exposure. This is collimation.

D True.

E False – Using an undercouch configuration the dose to the operator will be less.

KEY CONCEPT

PERSONAL PROTECTIVE EQUIPMENT

Personal protective equipment (PPE) provides protection from scattered radiation or primary radiation which has been transmitted through the patient. It does not provide protection against unattenuated primary radiation.

A2.21 THE FOLLOWING FACTORS INFLUENCE THE ENTRANCE SURFACE DOSE

A   True – This is because different image receptors require different amounts of radiation to produce an image.

B   True – As the ESD required will vary depending on how much is absorbed as it passes through the patient.

C   True.

D   True – This can be changed by altering the tube potential, kV waveform and tube filtration.

E   True – As radiation is absorbed by materials between the patient and the image receptor (anti-scatter grids, cassette faces, table tops) the exposure must be increased to compensate for this and hence increase the ESD.

A2.22 REGARDING GENERAL RADIATION PROTECTION PRINCIPLES

A   True.

B   False – The tube incorporates lead shielding to attenuate radiation.

C   False – Leakage radiation at 1 m from the focus should not exceed 1 mGy in one hour.

D   True.

E   False – The aim of radiation protection is to reduce stochastic and deterministic effects.

A2.23 GENERAL RADIATION PROTECTION

A   True.

B   False – Lead aprons do not provide protection from the primary beam or against high energy gamma radiation but do protect against radiation attenuated or scattered by the patient.

C   False – They are recommended to be worn during all procedures.

D   False – Lead aprons are normally 0.25 mm Pb equivalent, or 0.35 mm Pb equivalent for interventional procedures.

E   False – The operator should never place their hand in the primary beam.

A2.24 RADIATION PROTECTION OF STAFF AND MEMBERS OF THE PUBLIC

A False – When all the machinery is turned off the x-ray room is no longer a controlled area.

B True.

C True.

D False – Members of the public should not receive more than 1 mSv per year.

E True.

A2.25 ABSORBED DOSE

A False – Absorbed dose is measured in gray (Gy).

B True.

C True.

D False – It is the equivalent dose that takes into account the effectiveness of different types of radiation in the production of biological damage.

E True.

A2.26 EQUIVALENT DOSE

A False – It is the absorbed dose multiplied by a radiation weighting factor.

B False.

C True.

D True.

E True.

A2.27 EFFECTIVE DOSE

A False – Is measured in Sv.

B False – Is the product of the equivalent dose multiplied by a tissue weighting factor, summed for all organs and tissues in the body.

C True.

D False.

E False – The effective dose of a CXR is 0.02 mSv.

A2.28 THE TYPICAL EFFECTIVE DOSE FOR THE FOLLOWING PROCEDURES ARE

A True.

B True.

C True.

D False – CT Abdomen = 10 mSv.

E True.

KEY CONCEPT

ABSORBED, EQUIVALENT AND EFFECTIVE DOSE

- **Absorbed dose** = Energy deposited per unit mass to a medium by the incident radiation.
  Measured in (J/kg)
  Units = gray (Gy)
  1 Gy = 1 J/kg
- **Equivalent dose** = Absorbed dose x radiation weighting factor.
  This value measures the radiation dose to a tissue accounting for the type of radiation received and its effectiveness at producing biological damage.
  Units = sieverts (Sv)
- **Effective dose** = Equivalent dose x tissue weighting factor, summed for all organs and tissues in the body.
  This accounts for the difference in sensitivity of the tissues to radiation.
  Units = mSv.

RADIATION WEIGHTING FACTORS

Radiation	Radiation weighting factor	Biological damage
X-rays	1	Lowest
Gamma rays	1	
Beta particles	1	
Positrons	1	
Neutrons	5–20	
Alpha particles	20	Highest

TISSUE WEIGHTING FACTORS

Organ/Tissue	Tissue weighting factor
Skin	0.01
Bladder	0.05
Breast	0.05
Liver	0.05
Bone marrow	0.20

TYPICAL EFFECTIVE DOSES

Investigation	Dose (mSv)
PA CXR	0.02
Skull AP/Lat	0.06
AP pelvis	0.7
AXR	0.7
Lumbar spine	1
CT brain	2
IVU	2.5
Barium meal	3
Bone scan	3
Barium enema	7
CT abdomen	10
Thallium scan	20

KEY CONCEPT

KERMA, ENTRANCE SURFACE DOSE AND DOSE AREA PRODUCT

- **Kerma** = The **K**inetic **E**nergy of the secondary electrons **R**eleased per unit **MA**ss of the irradiated material
- **Entrance surface dose (ESD)** = Absorbed dose to air at the point of intersection of the x-ray beam axis with the entrance surface of the patient.
- **Dose area product (DAP)** = The absorbed dose to air averaged over the area of the x-ray beam perpendicular to the beam axis multiplied by the area of the beam in the same plane. Units = $Gy.cm^2$.

CHAPTER 3

General radiation protection

Q3.1 CONCERNING THERMOLUMINESCENT DOSIMETERS (TLD)

A   The chips cannot be reused.

B   They can distinguish radioactive contamination.

C   They require a filtered badge to provide energy discrimination.

D   They can record a wide range of dose.

E   They can provide a direct reading of personal dose.

Q3.2 CONCERNING FILM BADGES

A   They are cheap.

B   They are not able to identify type and energy of exposure.

C   They do not provide a permanent record of exposure.

D   They require a dark room and wet processing.

E   They are resistant to heat, humidity and chemicals.

Q3.3 CONCERNING ELECTRONIC PERSONAL DOSIMETERS (EPD)

A   They provide direct readings.

B   They are cheap.

C   They have a linear response to dose.

D   They record doses from 20 keV to 10 MeV.

E   They provide an audible warning of high dose rates.

Q3.4 REGARDING PERSONAL DOSIMETRY SYSTEMS

A   Personal monitoring film in a film badge is single coated.

B   A TLD contains a small chip of iron oxide mounted in a plastic holder.

C   To process a thermoluminescent chip it requires heating to approximately 400°C.

D   Electronic dosimeters have a poor response to photon energies below 80 keV.

E   Electronic personal dosimeters are 50–200 times more sensitive than a TLD.

Q3.5 REGARDING PERSONAL DOSIMETRY SYSTEMS

A   Film badges provide a permanent record of exposure.

B   Processing of a thermoluminescent personal dosimeter (TLD) requires cooling.

C   Thermoluminescent personal dosimeters cannot distinguish radioactive contamination.

D Electronic personal dosimeters (EPD) provide a direct reading ranging from 20 keV to 10 MeV.

E Film badges require calibration using a gamma source.

Q3.6 THE FOLLOWING ARE ADVANTAGES OF AN ELECTRONIC PERSONAL DOSIMETER

A Linear response to dose.

B Initial cost.

C Direct readings.

D Can record doses between 20 keV and 10 MeV.

E Measures personal dose directly at the skin and at depth.

Q3.7 THE FOLLOWING ARE ADVANTAGES OF A FILM DOSIMETER

A They are commonly used to measure patient dose.

B They are cheap.

C They provide an instantaneous read out.

D They are insensitive to humidity.

E They produce a permanent record of exposure.

Q3.8 THE FOLLOWING ARE DISADVANTAGES OF A TLD

A There is no permanent record of doses.

B They are less sensitive than film dosimeters.

C Do not provide an instantaneous record.

D Narrow dose range with an exponential response to dose.

E They are more expensive than film dosimeters.

Q3.9 CONCERNING DOSIMETERS AND THEIR MEDICAL APPLICATIONS

A TLD dosimeters are used to measure patient skin dose.

B TLDs are used for in-beam diagnostic x-ray measurements.

C Scintillators are used to measure contamination and environmental monitoring.

D Ionisation chambers are used in quality control measurements.

E Radiophotoluminescent dosimeters are used in personal dosimetry.

Q3.10 THE POTENTIAL EFFECTS OF HIGH DOSE RADIATION RECEIVED BY A FOETUS INCLUDE

A Intrauterine death.

B Immunosuppression.

C Growth retardation.

D Microcephaly.

E Childhood cancers.

Q3.11 THE BIOLOGICAL EFFECTS OF A HIGH RADIATION DOSE TO A FOETUS INCLUDE

A The development of leukaemia.

B Gross malformations.

C Sickle cell anaemia.

D Osteogenesis imperfecta.

E Reduced IQ.

Q3.12 THE POSSIBLE EFFECTS OF RADIATION TO AN EMBRYO OR FOETUS

A Are dependent on the radiation dose received and the stage in pregnancy.

B The most critical time for effects on the brain is between 8 and 15 weeks gestation.

C There is an increased risk of foetal death during organogenesis.

D There is increased risk of abnormal foetal development during the pre-implantation phase.

E The risk of inducing a childhood cancer is likely to be lower during the early stages of pregnancy.

Q3.13 CONCERNING EFFECTS TO A FOETUS FROM ANTENATAL EXPOSURE

A High doses (>100 mGy) are required to cause early death of an embryo.

B Cancer induction is a deterministic effect.

C The highest risk for mental retardation is during the third trimester.

D The foetus is vulnerable to a risk of cancer induction from conception.

E The cancer risk (number per 100 individuals exposed to 1 Sv) from *in utero* exposure up to the age of 15 years old is 10.

Answers

A3.1 CONCERNING THERMOLUMINESCENT DOSIMETERS (TLD)

A False – The chips can be reused, this is an advantage of a TLD.

B False – This is not possible.

C True.

D True – They can record doses between 0.1 mSv and 2000 mSv.

E True.

A3.2 CONCERNING FILM BADGES

A True.

B False – They are able to identify both the type of energy and exposure.

C False.

D True.

E False – This is a disadvantage of film badges.

A3.3 CONCERNING ELECTRONIC PERSONAL DOSIMETERS (EPD)

A True.

B False – The initial cost is expensive.

C True.

D True.

E True.

A3.4 REGARDING PERSONAL DOSIMETRY SYSTEMS

A False – The film is double coated, containing a slow and a fast emulsion.

B False – It contains a small chip of lithium fluoride.

C True – This causes the trapped electrons to be released and fall to their ground state emitting photons of light.

D True.

E True.

A3.5 REGARDING PERSONAL DOSIMETRY SYSTEMS

A True – They can detect a wide range of doses from 0.1 mSv to 1000 mSv.

B False – TLDs require heating to release the trapped electrons.

C True.

D True.

E True.

A3.6 THE FOLLOWING ARE ADVANTAGES OF AN ELECTRONIC PERSONAL DOSIMETER

A True.

B False – These are expensive to buy initially; this is a disadvantage.

C True.

D True.

E True.

A3.7 THE FOLLOWING ARE ADVANTAGES OF A FILM DOSIMETER

A False.

B True.

C False – They do not provide an instantaneous read out, this is a disadvantage.

D False – They are sensitive to heat and humidity; this is a disadvantage.

E True.

A3.8 THE FOLLOWING ARE DISADVANTAGES OF TLDS

A True.

B False – They are slightly more sensitive than film dosimeters.

C True.

D False – TLDs have a wide dose range with a linear response to dose; this is an advantage.

E True.

A3.9 CONCERNING DOSIMETERS AND THEIR MEDICAL APPLICATIONS

A True.

B False – Ionisation chambers are used to measure this as part of quality control.

C True.

D True.

E True.

A3.10 THE POTENTIAL EFFECTS OF HIGH DOSE RADIATION RECEIVED BY A FOETUS INCLUDE

A True – This occurs as result of exposure in early pregnancy.

B False.

C True.

D True.

E True.

A3.11 THE BIOLOGICAL EFFECTS OF A HIGH RADIATION DOSE TO A FOETUS INCLUDE

A True.

B True.

C False.

D False.

E True.

A3.12 THE POSSIBLE EFFECTS OF RADIATION TO AN EMBRYO OR FOETUS

A True.

B True.

C False – The risk of foetal death is highest during the pre-implantation period.

D False – There is an increased risk of abnormal foetal development during organogenesis.

E True.

A3.13 CONCERNING EFFECTS TO A FOETUS FROM ANTENATAL EXPOSURE

A   True – This is a deterministic effect; a dose threshold exists.

B   False – This is a stochastic effect; no dose threshold exists.

C   False.

D   False – The foetus is vulnerable from three weeks *in utero*.

E   False – The risk of a fatal cancer is 3 per 100 individuals exposed per sievert.

KEY CONCEPT

THE EFFECTS OF RADIATION ON THE FOETUS

The possible effects of a high radiation dose received by an embryo or foetus are dependent on both the magnitude of the radiation dose and the stage of pregnancy.

Procedure	Foetal dose	Risk of childhood cancer
CXR	< 0.01 mGy	Negligible
Chest CT	0.06 mGy	Minimal
Pelvic x-ray	1.1 mGy	Very low
AXR	1.4 mGy	Very low
Barium enema	7 mGy	Low
Pelvic CT	25 mGy	Low

CHAPTER 4

Ionising Radiation Regulations 1999

Q4.1 IN THE IONISING RADIATION REGULATIONS 1999 (IRR 99), REGARDING RADIATION SAFETY

A The employer must provide personal protective equipment.

B For pregnant employees, the equivalent dose received by the foetus should not exceed 10 mSv during the pregnancy.

C The employer must ensure a critical examination of new x-ray equipment is performed.

D Dose limits are not exceeded.

E A regular quality assurance programme for x-ray equipment is performed.

Q4.2 CONCERNING IRR 99

A The aim is to protect patients from ionising radiation.

B The enforcing authority is the Health and Safety Executive (HSE).

C The employer is responsible for employing a Radiation Protection Advisor (RPA).

D Local rules are required for controlled areas and may be provided for supervised areas.

E The RPA is consulted on requirements for controlled and supervised areas.

Q4.3 REGARDING IRR 99

A The regulations are enforced by the Chief Executive.

B The aim is to ensure that the radiation dose received by patients is kept as low as reasonably practicable.

C They apply to the radiation protection of staff, members of the public and some equipment aspects of patient protection.

D The employer is the main duty holder and must ensure that the requirements of the regulations are carried out.

E IRR are supported by an ACoP (Approved Code of Practice) which provides practical advice on how to comply with the law.

Q4.4 THE ROLE OF A RADIATION PROTECTION ADVISOR INCLUDES

A The designation of controlled and supervised areas.

B Drawing up and supervising the arrangements set out in the local rules.

C   Calibration of monitoring equipment.

D   Planning of installations and acceptance of equipment.

E   Quality assurance programmes.

Q4.5 A DOSE CONSTRAINT

A   Is used to restrict exposure to ionising radiation.

B   Is a dose limit of radiation exposure, above which an investigation must be instigated.

C   Does not apply in the context of comforters and carers.

D   Is an upper level of individual dose specified by the employer at the design or planning stage.

E   Should represent a level of dose which should be achievable in a well managed practice.

Q4.6 A CONTROLLED AREA

A   Is required if any individual working in the area is likely to receive an effective dose greater than 3 mSv.

B   Must have a warning sign at the entrance.

C   Is required if a working individual will receive an equivalent dose more than 10% of any relevant dose limit.

D   Includes the radiopharmacy.

E   Is required to restrict significant radiation exposure above specified levels defined by physical boundaries.

Q4.7 REGARDING DESIGNATED AREAS

A A controlled area must be designated if any individual working within the area is likely to receive an equivalent dose greater than 6 mSv or an effective dose greater than three-tenths of any relevant dose limit.

B A supervised area must be designated if an employee is likely to receive an equivalent dose greater than 1 mSv per year or an effective dose greater than one-tenth of any relevant dose limit.

C These should be monitored to ensure that the levels of ionising radiation are appropriate.

D Local rules are applied to all controlled areas.

E These areas have special procedures that are necessary to restrict the possibility of significant exposure.

Q4.8 REGARDING CONTROLLED AREAS

A They are required if any worker is likely to receive an effective dose of more than 3 mSv per annum.

B Around a mobile x-ray set is determined by the operator which extends 2 m around the x-ray tube and patient.

C There must be set local rules.

D Has similar dose limits to a supervised area.

E This includes areas where the dose rate averaged over one minute is greater than 7.5 µSv per hour.

Q4.9 A SUPERVISED AREA

A Is an area in which any individual is likely to receive an effective dose of more than 2 mSv per year.

B Is an area monitored to ensure radiation doses are kept within certain limits.

C   Has no set local rules.

D   Can become a controlled area if dose limits are exceeded.

E   Is an area in which any individual is likely to receive an effective dose greater than one-tenth of a relevant dose limit.

Q4.10 REGARDING SUPERVISED AREAS

A   These areas should be 'signed' where appropriate.

B   Has dose rates which are less than those in a controlled area.

C   Has a Radiation Protection Advisor (RPA) appointed to monitor adherence to the local rules.

D   A Radiation Protection Supervisor (RPS) must be consulted on the designation of areas.

E   Records of radiation levels in designated areas must be kept.

Q4.11 CONCERNING CLASSIFIED WORKERS

A   An individual who receives an equivalent dose of more than 6 mSv per annum must be designated as a classified worker.

B   The total annual effective dose limit of a classified worker is 20 mSv.

C   An employee under the age of 18 requires special permission to become a classified worker.

D   An employee who receives more than three-tenths (30%) of any other dose limit should be classified.

E   Medical surveillance of a classified worker is only necessary if the annual effective dose limit is exceeded.

Q4.12 REGARDING CLASSIFIED WORKERS

A All radiation dose records are submitted to a Central Index of Dose Information, operated for the HSE.

B Personal monitoring of the radiation dose received is not mandatory.

C The annual effective dose limit of classified workers is 6 mSv.

D The records of classified workers must be kept until the individual is 50 years old or for at least 30 years.

E The employee must be declared fit prior to being designated a classified worker.

Q4.13 REGARDING DOSE LIMITS

A The effective dose limit per annum is the same for all employees.

B The effective dose to an extremity must not exceed 500 mSv.

C The dose limit to a foetus should be less than 1 mSv throughout the whole pregnancy.

D If the annual dose limit is exceeded in an employee under the age of 18 they should become a classified worker.

E The equivalent dose to the skin should not exceed 500 mSv for a classified worker.

Q4.14 CONCERNING DOSE LIMITS

A A female of reproductive age should not receive more than 13 mSv in any consecutive three months.

B The equivalent dose limit to the eye in an individual under the age of 18 should not exceed 50 mSv.

C The effective dose limit per annum for a member of the public is 0.1 mSv.

D The effective dose limit for employees aged over 18 years is 20 mSv per year.

E The dose limits for extremities, skin and the eye are stated in terms of effective dose.

Q4.15 CONCERNING DOSE LIMITS

A For employees over 18 years of age the limit on equivalent dose for the lens of the eye is 150 mSv per year.

B For employees over 18 years of age the limit on equivalent dose to the extremities is 500 mSv per year.

C For trainees less than 18 years of age the limit on effective dose is 6 mSv per year.

D The limit of equivalent dose for the abdomen of any woman of reproductive capacity is 13 mSv in any three consecutive months.

E The limit of effective dose for any person other than an employee or trainee is 1 mSv per year.

Q4.16 FORMAL INVESTIGATION LEVELS FOR WORKERS

A Are determined locally.

B Are set following advice from the RPS.

C Must be specified in the local rules.

D Are the same as dose constraints.

E Are necessary to instigate a review of working conditions if the dose is exceeded.

Q4.17 CONCERNING OVEREXPOSURES

A Notification should occur if a patient receives more than 10 times the intended dose for a skull x-ray.

B The threshold for reporting an overexposure of a CXR is 20 times the intended dose.

C Incidents should be reported if the medical exposure is much greater than intended.

D Patients should not be informed about the incident until it has been investigated.

E If due to faulty equipment the machine should be used with extreme caution.

Q4.18 REGARDING OVEREXPOSURES

A The Radiation Protection Advisor (RPA), who will provide advice on further action, should be informed.

B The dose received by the patient should be calculated.

C Near misses should be reported to the Health and Safety Executive (HSE).

D All spillages of radioactive material must be reported to the Health Care Commission.

E A record of the incident should be kept for a minimum of six years.

Q4.19 THE FOLLOWING INCIDENTS SHOULD BE REPORTED IF A PATIENT RECEIVES

A 1.2 times the intended dose during radionuclide therapy.

B 3 times the intended dose for a mammogram.

C   1.5 times the intended dose for an IVU.

D   10 times the dose for an abdominal x-ray.

E   10 times the intended dose for a skull x-ray.

Q4.20 CONCERNING DOSE CONSTRAINTS FOR COMFORTERS AND CARERS

A   The use of supporting devices and restraining equipment is sometimes necessary to hold a child in position during radiography.

B   A parent can comfort a child if adequately protected from the x-rays.

C   A parent is protected from the primary beam as long as they are wearing a lead apron.

D   A TLD can be worn by the comforter to provide a direct reading of the dose received.

E   The comforter should be positioned outside of the primary beam.

Q4.21 A QUALITY ASSURANCE PROGRAMME

A   Is necessary to comply with both IRR 99 and IR(ME)R regulations.

B   Provides essential accurate records that the equipment was functioning properly in the event of an incident.

C   Ensures that the best quality radiographs are produced at the first attempt at an acceptable radiation dose.

D   Is performed by a radiologist.

E   Involves two levels of tests.

Q4.22 THE FOLLOWING ASPECTS OF PERFORMANCE OF AN X-RAY MACHINE ARE TESTED

A The focal spot.

B Accuracy and consistency of the kV.

C The alignment of the x-ray beam and the bucky.

D Automatic Enlargement Control.

E Leakage of radiation through the tube housing.

Q4.23 THE FOLLOWING EQUIPMENT IS USED IN QUALITY ASSURANCE TESTING

A An ionisation chamber.

B Pinhole test object.

C Star test objects.

D A densitometer.

E A sensitometer.

Q4.24 REGARDING EQUIPMENT QUALITY ASSURANCE

A It aims to ensure the production of optimum quality images with the least dose to the patient.

B It involves rigorous and regular checks over the lifetime of the imaging equipment.

C The critical examination is completed by the installer in conjunction with the Radiation Protection Supervisor.

D Routine performance testing is undertaken on a regular basis.

E Under IRR 99 the Chief Executive can be held personally liable.

Q4.25 BASIC QUALITY ASSURANCE MEASUREMENTS FOR X-RAY TUBES INCLUDE

A Focal spot size.

B Light beam to x-ray field alignment.

C Personal protective equipment.

D Applied kV calibration.

E Automatic exposure control consistency.

Q4.26 CONCERNING QUALITY ASSURANCE ON ANCILLARY EQUIPMENT

A The quality assurance of image intensifiers is usually performed using a manufacturer's QC phantom.

B The Huttner test object is used to assess the spatial resolution of the image intensifier.

C Leeds test objects are black discs containing various items which show on the intensifier television system.

D Leeds test objects are so called because they were developed at the University of Leeds.

E Quality assurance tests on image intensifiers only need to be performed every 10 years.

Answers

A4.1 IN THE IONISING RADIATION REGULATIONS 1999 (IRR 99), REGARDING RADIATION SAFETY

A True – Storage facilities for this equipment and regular examinations must be performed to ensure proper maintenance.

B False – After the employer has been notified, the equivalent dose to the foetus should not exceed 1 mSv for the remainder of the pregnancy.

C False – The installer is responsible for the critical examination of new equipment.

D True.

E True – This is the responsibility of the employer.

A4.2 CONCERNING IRR 99

A False – The IRR aims to minimise radiation exposure to employees and members of the public.

B True.

C True.

D True.

E True.

A4.3 REGARDING IRR 99

A False – The regulations are enforced by the Health and Safety Executive.

B False – They aim to ensure that the exposure of ionising radiation to employees and members of the public is as low as reasonably practicable (ALARP).

C True.

D True.

E True.

A4.4 THE ROLE OF A RADIATION PROTECTION ADVISOR INCLUDES

A True.

B False – The RPA will draw up the local rules and contingency plans but the Radiation Protection Supervisor (RPS) oversees the arrangements set out in the local rules.

C True.

D True.

E True.

A4.5 A DOSE CONSTRAINT

A True.

B False – It is not a dose limit or investigation level but a dose level which should be achievable in a well managed department.

C False.

D True.

E True.

A4.6 A CONTROLLED AREA

A False – A controlled area is defined as an area in which any individual is likely to receive an effective dose greater than 6 mSv.

B True.

C False – It is an equivalent dose more than 30% of any relevant dose limit.

D True.

E True.

A4.7 REGARDING DESIGNATED AREAS

A False.

B False.

C True.

D True.

E True.

A4.8 REGARDING CONTROLLED AREAS

A False – Are required if any individual receives more than 6 mSv a year.

B True.

C True.

D False.

E True.

A4.9 A SUPERVISED AREA

A False – Likely to receive a dose of more than 1 mSv per year.

B True.

C False – Local rules are written where appropriate and monitored by a Radiation Protection Supervisor.

D True.

E False – If an individual receives an *equivalent dose* of more than one-tenth of a relevant dose limit it should be designated a controlled area.

A4.10 REGARDING SUPERVISED AREAS

A True.

B True.

C False – A Radiation Protection Supervisor has this role.

D False – This is the role of the RPA.

E True.

A4.11 CONCERNING CLASSIFIED WORKERS

A False – An employee who exceeds an *effective dose* of more than 6 mSv per year should become classified.

B True.

C False – No individual under 18 years of age can become a classified worker.

D True.

E False – Health and radiation monitoring are statutory.

KEY CONCEPT

CONTROLLED AND SUPERVISED AREAS

A **controlled area** is designated so that special working procedures are in place to protect individuals from excessive radiation above set parameters. It is also designed to limit the probability and magnitude of accidents.

These limits are as follows.

- Any person working in the area likely to receive an effective dose of more than 6 mSv per annum.
- Any person working in the area likely to receive an equivalent dose greater than three-tenths (30%) of any relevant dose limit.
- Areas where the dose rate averaged over one minute exceeds 7.5 μSv per hour and untrained employees may enter. This was added by the ACoP (Approved Code of Practice).
- Any area where there is significant risk of spread of contamination.

A **supervised area** is an area of monitoring only. It is necessary to keep conditions under review as if set limits are exceeded it should be designated a controlled area. These limits are as follows.

- Any individual likely to receive an effective dose of more than 1 mSv per annum.
- Any individual likely to receive an equivalent dose greater than one-tenth (10%) of a relevant dose limit.

A4.12 REGARDING CLASSIFIED WORKERS

A True.

B False – Personal monitoring is a requirement of a classified worker.

C False – This is the annual effective dose limit for non-classified workers.

D False – Records must be kept until the individual is (or would be) 75 years of age or for at least 50 years.

E True – An appointed doctor must deem the employee to be fit prior to designation.

KEY CONCEPT

CLASSIFIED WORKERS

- Annual effective dose limit is 20 mSv.
- Employees who receive an effective dose of more than 6 mSv must be classified.
- Employees who receive an equivalent dose of more than three-tenths (30%) of any relevant dose limit should be classified.
- No individual under the age of 18 can become a classified worker.
- Health and radiation monitoring is mandatory.
- Records of dose assessments must be kept until the employee is 75 or for at least 50 years.

A4.13 REGARDING DOSE LIMITS

A False – There are reduced dose limits for employees less than 18 years of age.

B False – The *equivalent dose* to an extremity should not exceed 500 mSv.

C True.

D False – No employee under the age of 18 can become a classified worker.

E True.

A4.14 CONCERNING DOSE LIMITS

A True.

B True.

C False – The effective dose limit is 1 mSv per annum.

D True.

E False – These are stated in terms of equivalent dose.

A4.15 CONCERNING DOSE LIMITS

A True.

B True.

C True.

D True.

E True.

A4.16 FORMAL INVESTIGATION LEVELS FOR WORKERS

A   True.

B   False – Are set following the advice from the RPA.

C   True.

D   False – A dose constraint is a level of dose which should be achievable in a well managed practice.

E   True – Legally an investigation must be carried out when an employee receives more than 15 mSv for the first time in any year.

A4.17 CONCERNING OVEREXPOSURES

A   False – Notification requires 20 times the intended dose.

B   True.

C   True.

D   False – Unless there is a good reason the individual should be informed immediately.

E   False – If due to faulty equipment it should be withdrawn from use and not returned until the fault has been investigated and rectified.

KEY CONCEPT

ANNUAL DOSE LIMITS (IRR 99)

Dose limits	Classified workers Age > 18	Non-classified workers	Others
Effective dose per year (mSv)	20	6	1
Equivalent dose to the lens of the eye (mSv)	150	50	15
Equivalent dose to an extremity (mSv)	500	150	50
Equivalent dose to the skin (mSv)	500	150	50

A4.18 REGARDING OVEREXPOSURES

A True.

B True.

C False – Near misses may require internal investigation only.

D False – Only spillages resulting in significant contamination need to be reported to the HSE.

E True.

A4.19 THE FOLLOWING INCIDENTS SHOULD BE REPORTED IF A PATIENT RECEIVES

A True.

B False – 10 times the intended dose should be reported.

C True.

D True.

E False – 20 times the intended dose should be reported.

A4.20 CONCERNING DOSE CONSTRAINTS FOR COMFORTERS AND CARERS

A True.

B True – This would not be recommended if the mother was pregnant.

C False – The parent should not be directly in the primary beam. The lead apron protects against scattered radiation.

KEY CONCEPT

NOTIFICATION OF INCIDENTS – IRR 99

- When extremity, skull, chest or dental x-rays are more than 20 times the intended dose.
- When an x-ray of the lumbar spine, abdomen or pelvis is 10 times the intended dose.
- If a mammogram exceeds 10 times the intended dose.
- If a barium enema, barium meal, IVU, angiogram or CT exceeds 1.5 times the intended dose limit.
- If there is spillage of a radioactive material which has resulted in significant contamination.
- Loss or theft of a radioactive source.

D False – An electronic personal dosimeter can be worn to provide a direct reading and reassure the comforter.

E True – They must also be protected by appropriate equipment or shielding.

A4.21 A QUALITY ASSURANCE PROGRAMME

A True – Both sets of regulations contain requirements relating to a quality assurance programme.

B True.

C True.

D False – These tests are usually performed by the equipment user, medical physics department or the medical engineers.

E True – The QA tests are divided into level A and level B tests.

A4.22 THE FOLLOWING ASPECTS OF PERFORMANCE OF AN X-RAY MACHINE ARE TESTED

A True.

B True.

C True.

D False – Automatic Exposure Control.

E True.

KEY CONCEPT

QUALITY ASSURANCE

Quality assurance is defined as the planned and systematic actions necessary to provide adequate confidence that a product or service will satisfy given requirements for quality.

Quality assurance tests

Level A	Level B
Quick and simple	Take longer
Require simple equipment	Require more complex analysis
Do not need detailed analysis	Requires detailed analysis
Performed frequently	Performed less than level A tests
Performed by the equipment user	Often performed by medical physicists

A4.23 THE FOLLOWING EQUIPMENT IS USED IN QUALITY ASSURANCE TESTING

A True.

B True.

C True.

D True.

E True.

A4.24 REGARDING EQUIPMENT QUALITY ASSURANCE

A True.

B True – These include a 'critical examination', 'acceptance test', 'commissioning test' and 'routine performance tests'.

C False – This is performed by the installer and the Radiation Protection Advisor (RPA).

D True – The time interval may vary depending on the equipment being tested.

E True.

A4.25 BASIC QUALITY ASSURANCE MEASUREMENTS FOR X-RAY TUBES INCLUDE

A True.

B True.

C False – This is not part of the x-ray tube.

D True.

E True.

A4.26 CONCERNING QUALITY ASSURANCE ON ANCILLARY EQUIPMENT

A False – These tests are usually performed with a set of 'Leeds' test objects.

B True.

C True – These are used to test image quality and requires the subjective assessment of images of various test objects.

D True.

E False – These tests are performed annually.

KEY CONCEPT

BASIC QUALITY ASSURANCE MEASUREMENTS

Basic measurement	Equipment
Applied kV calibration	Keithley divider
	Electronic penetrameter
X-ray output	Ionisation chamber
	Electrometer
Light beam to x-ray field alignment	Film
	Phantom/wires
Focal spot size	Gold/platinum alloy pinhole
	Star resolution grid
Total tube filtration	Ionisation chamber
	Electrometer
Timer	Spinning top
	Electronic timing device
Tube housing leakage	Films in cassettes
	Ionisation chamber
	Electrometer
Automatic Exposure Control	Films in cassettes
	Densitometer
	Ionisation chamber/electrometer
Protective clothing	Visual inspection of gloves and aprons
	Radiographic examination

.

CHAPTER 5

Ionising Radiation (Medical Exposure) Regulations 2000

Q5.1 IR(ME)R 2000 APPLIES TO THE EXPOSURE OF

A Patients undergoing medical diagnosis or treatment.

B Individuals as part of an occupational health survey.

C Individuals as part of medico-legal procedures.

D Individuals participating in medical research programmes.

E Individuals as part of health screening.

Q5.2 REGARDING IR(ME)R 2000 REQUIREMENTS

A An individual under the age of 16 is considered a child in England and Wales.

B An individual under the age of 18 is considered a child in Scotland.

C Emigration chest x-rays are not included within the scope of medico-legal exposures.

D Applies to the exposure of patients as part of their own medical diagnosis or treatment.

E A framework for protection of the patient is provided by the employer's written procedures.

Q5.3 UNDER THE IR(ME)(A)R 2006

A *Practitioner* means a registered healthcare professional who is entitled to refer individuals for medical exposure to a radiologist.

B *Referrer* means a registered healthcare professional who is entitled to take responsibility for an individual exposure.

C The duty of the employer is to investigate incidents and report to the Department of Health if appropriate.

D The enforcing authority in England is the Secretary of State for Health.

E The exposure of individuals as part of medico-legal procedures is no longer included in the regulations.

Q5.4 UNDER IR(ME)R 2000 THE DUTIES OF AN EMPLOYER INCLUDE

A To ensure that practitioners and operators are trained and undertake continued professional development.

B To investigate incidents of overexposure and report to the Healthcare Commission if appropriate.

C   To establish diagnostic reference levels.

D   To produce written protocols.

E   To establish quality assurance programmes for the procedures.

Q5.5 REGARDING THE DUTIES OF A PRACTITIONER, OPERATOR AND REFERRER

A   A referrer will be responsible for justification.

B   Only radiographers and radiologists may act as operators.

C   Radiographers may act as practitioners.

D   The only requirement on the referrer is to provide adequate relevant clinical information.

E   Individual duty holders can be prosecuted under IR(ME)R.

Q5.6 CONCERNING INCIDENT REPORTING

A   IR(ME)R requires the employer to report all incidents which exceed the diagnostic reference level.

B   If a patient receives 10 times the intended dose for a chest x-ray the incident should be notified.

C   If the intended dose of a barium enema is exceeded by three times the incident should be notified.

D   The employer must inform the Department of Health if an individual is exposed to ionising radiation to an extent much greater than intended.

E   Patients who have received a dose much greater than intended should be informed of the incident.

Q5.7 CONCERNING RADIATION PROTECTION

A   Justification ensures that the difference between benefit and harm is maximised.

B   CT only requires justification for high dose procedures.

C   Optimisation ensures that we undertake the practice to maximise the difference between benefit and harm.

D   Optimisation involves giving the required dose to obtain the best image quality.

E   Optimisation is achieving adequate image quality at the lowest possible dose.

Q5.8 THE ROLE OF A MEDICAL PHYSICS EXPERT INCLUDES

A   Consultation on the justification of a radiological procedure.

B   Consultation on optimisation including patient dosimetry and quality assurance.

C   Provision of advice on matters relating to radiation protection concerning medical exposures.

D   Monitoring adherence to local rules.

E   The ability to act as an operator in certain circumstances.

Q5.9 REGARDING JUSTIFICATION OF AN INDIVIDUAL EXPOSURE THE FOLLOWING MUST BE CONSIDERED

A   The specific objectives of the exposure.

B   The total diagnostic or therapeutic benefit.

C   The individual detriment that the exposure may cause.

D   Whether an alternative technique can be used which may provide less exposure to ionising radiation.

E   The urgency of the radiological procedure.

Q5.10 OPTIMISATION OF A RADIOLOGICAL PROCEDURE INCLUDES

A   Keeping doses as low as reasonably practicable (ALARP) in most cases.

B   Ensuring doses to non-target volumes and tissues must be ALARP.

C   The operator must pay attention to the diagnostic reference levels.

D   Not all medical exposures require clinical evaluation.

E   Set departmental policies established to reduce patient dose.

Q5.11 OPTIMISATION INCLUDES

A   Quality assurance.

B   Assessment of dose.

C   Adherence to diagnostic reference levels.

D   Information for nuclear medicine patients, their comforters and carers.

E   Research procedures.

Q5.12 CONCERNING EXPOSURES DURING PREGNANCY

A All females between the ages of 16 to 55 years should be asked if they could be pregnant.

B Where foetal doses are in excess of 50 mGy there is a substantial chance of growth retardation and central nervous system damage.

C A CT examination of a pregnant patient cannot be justified.

D An abdominal x-ray would provide a mean foetal dose of 1.4 mGy having a probability of 1 in 24000 of developing a fatal cancer in childhood.

E Exposures during the third trimester can lead to gross malformations.

Q5.13 CONCERNING IDENTIFICATION OF PATIENTS

A Female patients between the ages of 12 and 55 years should be asked about the possibility of pregnancy.

B Trainees are unable to identify patients.

C A record of identification must be made.

D The individual who identifies the patient must follow a standard identification protocol.

E There are set procedures to correctly identify an individual to be exposed.

Q5.14 REGARDING DOSE RECORDING AND DIAGNOSTIC REFERENCE LEVELS

A Adequate details should be kept of each procedure to enable assessments of patient dose.

B Local diagnostic reference levels are set by the Radiation Protection Supervisor.

C   The local diagnostic reference levels are always the same as the national DRLs.

D   The employer must investigate if a dose reference level is exceeded.

E   The entrance surface dose of a procedure can be estimated from measurements using an ionisation chamber.

Q5.15 CONCERNING DOSE RECORDING

A   Entrance surface dose is measured using an ionisation chamber or thermoluminescent dosimeter.

B   Dose area product is measured in mGy.

C   In nuclear medicine administered activity is measured using the dose length product.

D   Screening times are recorded in seconds.

E   The entrance surface dose is measured in $mGy.cm^2$.

Q5.16 CONCERNING DIAGNOSTIC REFERENCE LEVELS

A   This is a dose limit set for each diagnostic procedure.

B   These set dose limits are the same in every hospital for a specific examination.

C   These can be assessed using the entrance surface dose, kV, mAs, DAP, or screening times.

D   For a barium enema is 5 mSv.

E   If exceeded the Department of Health must be informed.

Q5.17 THE FOLLOWING ARE TRUE REGARDING TRAINING UNDER IR(ME)R 2000

A   An operator cannot carry out any practical aspect of a medical exposure without adequate training.

B   A trainee may not participate in practical aspects of a procedure.

C   A relevant certificate is sufficient proof of training.

D   The employer must keep training records.

E   Trainees may only observe procedures.

Q5.18 CONCERNING RESEARCH EXPOSURES

A   There is no dose constraint for individuals participating in research.

B   Individuals participating in research must be advised of the risk of exposure.

C   Voluntary consent must be obtained.

D   Research exposures are not included under the IR(ME)R guidelines.

E   There are set doses for individuals for whom no direct medical benefit is expected.

Answers

A5.1 IR(ME)R 2000 APPLIES TO THE EXPOSURE OF

A True.

B True.

C True.

D True.

E True.

A5.2 REGARDING IR(ME)R 2000 REQUIREMENTS

A False – An individual under the age of 18 is considered a child in England and Wales.

B False – An individual under the age of 16 is considered a child in Scotland.

C False – IR(ME)R applies to the exposure of individuals as part of medico-legal procedures.

D True.

E True.

A5.3 UNDER THE IR(ME)(A)R 2006

A False.

B False.

C False.

D False.

E False.

KEY CONCEPT

IR(ME)(A)R 2006

Amendments were made to the Ionising Radiation (Medical Exposure) Regulations 2000 which came into force from 1 November 2006. These are known as Ionising Radiation (Medical Exposure) (Amendment) Regulations 2006. IR(ME)(A)R.

These amendments include the following.

- *Practitioner* means a registered healthcare professional (previously registered medical practitioner) who is entitled in accordance with the employer's procedures to take responsibility for an individual exposure.
- *Referrer* means a registered healthcare professional (previously registered medical practitioner) who is entitled in accordance with the employer's procedures to refer individuals for medical exposure to a practitioner.
- The duty of the employer is to investigate incidents and report to the Healthcare Commission (previously the responsibility of the Department of Health).
- The enforcing authority in England is the Commission for Healthcare, Audit and Inspection – known as the Healthcare Commission (previously the responsibility of the Secretary of State for Health).

A5.4 UNDER IR(ME)R 2000 THE DUTIES OF AN EMPLOYER INCLUDE

A True.

B False – Under IR(ME)R 2000 incidents were reported to the Department of Health; IR(ME)(A)R changed this to the Healthcare Commission.

C True.

D True.

E True.

A5.5 REGARDING THE DUTIES OF A PRACTITIONER, OPERATOR AND REFERRER

A False – The practitioner is responsible for justification.

B False.

C   True.

D   False – Referrers must also supply patient ID information, their unique signature and LMP.

E   True.

A5.6 CONCERNING INCIDENT REPORTING

A   False – Only incidents where individuals are exposed to ionising radiation to an extent much greater than intended should be reported.

B   False – The employer must notify the incident if a patient receives 20 times the intended dose for a chest x-ray.

C   True.

D   False – Incidents are reported to the Healthcare Commission.

E   True – Unless there is a good reason for not doing so, individuals should be informed.

A5.7 CONCERNING RADIATION PROTECTION

A   False – This is optimisation.

B   False – All CT procedures require justification.

C   True.

D   False – Optimisation involves achieving adequate images at the lowest possible dose.

E   True.

A5.8 THE ROLE OF A MEDICAL PHYSICS EXPERT INCLUDES

A   False – Justification of a medical exposure is carried out by a practitioner.

B   True.

C   True.

D   False – This is a role of the Radiation Protection Supervisor.

E   True – An operator is anyone who carries out a practical aspect of the exposure.

A5.9 REGARDING JUSTIFICATION OF AN INDIVIDUAL EXPOSURE THE FOLLOWING MUST BE CONSIDERED

A True.

B True.

C True.

D True.

E True.

A5.10 OPTIMISATION OF A RADIOLOGICAL PROCEDURE INCLUDES

A False – All exposures must be kept ALARP.

B True.

C True.

D False – All procedures require clinical evaluation.

E True.

A5.11 OPTIMISATION INCLUDES

A True – This ensures all procedures are regularly reviewed and identifies any necessary amendments.

B True – To ensure doses are kept ALARP.

C True.

D True – This must specify how doses to other persons can be restricted as far as reasonably possible.

E True – Where there is no direct benefit to the individual the dose constraint is adhered to.

A5.12 CONCERNING EXPOSURES DURING PREGNANCY

A False – Pregnancy enquiries should include patients aged 12 to 55 years.

B False – Foetal doses in excess of 500 mGy can cause growth retardation and CNS damage.

C False – The benefit of the examination must justify the risk.

D True.

E False – This tends to occur from exposure in the first trimester.

KEY CONCEPT

THE ROLES OF DUTY HOLDERS UNDER IR(ME)R 2000

- Employer – to provide a framework of radiation protection.
- Practitioner – to justify each individual medical exposure.
- Operator – to undertake medical exposure or any work influencing exposure (e.g. calibration). They also have the responsibility for optimisation.
- Referrer – to provide the practitioner with sufficient clinical information for the justification process.
- Justification – the risk of the procedure is outweighed by the benefit.
- Optimisation – to ensure the patient receives the benefit from an exposure with the minimum risk.

A5.13 CONCERNING IDENTIFICATION OF PATIENTS

A   True.

B   False – Trainees can participate in any practical aspect of the procedure if they are adequately supervised.

C   True.

D   True.

E   True.

A5.14 REGARDING DOSE RECORDING AND DIAGNOSTIC REFERENCE LEVELS

A   True.

B   False – These DRLs are set by the employer.

C   False.

D   False – An investigation must take place if a dose reference level is consistently exceeded.

E   True.

A5.15 CONCERNING DOSE RECORDING

A True.

B False – DAP is measured using a DAP meter; the units are Gy.cm^2.

C False – Administered activity is measured using an isotope calibrator; the units are MBq.

D True.

E False – ESD is measured in Gy.

A5.16 CONCERNING DIAGNOSTIC REFERENCE LEVELS

A False – DRLs are dose levels or amounts of radioactivity used in a diagnostic procedure for typical examinations. It is not a dose limit.

B False – Each hospital sets its own DRLs for a given examination.

C True.

D False – The DRLs are in readily measurable quantities such as DAP or screening times.

E False.

A5.17 THE FOLLOWING ARE TRUE REGARDING TRAINING UNDER IR(ME)R 2000

A True.

B False – A trainee can participate in a practical aspect of a procedure if they are adequately supervised by a trained individual.

C True.

D True.

E False.

A5.18 CONCERNING RESEARCH EXPOSURES

A False – Dose constraints are set and adhered to.

B True – Individuals are advised of the risks in advance.

C True.

D False.

E True.

CHAPTER 6

X-ray production

Q6.1 CONCERNING THE PRODUCTION OF X-RAY PHOTONS FROM AN X-RAY TUBE

A   The filament voltage is responsible for accelerating the electrons towards the target.

B   After being accelerated the electrons bombard the negative anode target.

C   The tube voltage is responsible for the energy of the emitted x-ray photons.

D   The tube current is responsible for the quantity of accelerated electrons.

E   The tube is filled with krypton gas to improve efficiency of x-ray production.

Q6.2 ACCELERATED ELECTRONS IN AN X-RAY TUBE

A May reach speeds of up to half the speed of light.

B Upon striking the anode the electron's energy is predominantly converted into heat rather than x-rays in a ratio of 10:1.

C Can be increased in number by increasing the filament voltage.

D If accelerated by a 100 kV tube potential may produce K shell characteristic radiation upon striking a tungsten anode.

E Can escape the tube envelope, which is why insulated housing is required.

Q6.3 CONCERNING HEAT REMOVAL FROM AN X-RAY TUBE

A The molybdenum stem of the anode is highly heat conductive to allow removal of heat from the anode disc.

B CT and fluoroscopic equipment have active heat removal systems as the tube may be utilised for long periods of time.

C The x-ray tube is surrounded by a cooling water bath.

D The main method of heat removal is by radiation and convection.

E The anode disc can store heat energy.

Q6.4 CONCERNING HIGH VOLTAGE GENERATORS

A A self-rectifying generator produces a constant kV.

B Full wave rectification inverts the negative component of the alternating voltage waveform into the positive component.

C Three phase generators enable the kVp to be at or near its maximum at all times.

D   For the same length of exposure a self-rectifying generator will be at its peak kVp for longer than a full wave rectified generator with the same kVp.

E   High frequency generators produce a virtually constant kVp.

Q6.5 CONCERNING CHARACTERISTIC RADIATION

A   It can be produced by the ejection of an electron from any shell.

B   The bombarding electrons need to have energy greater than the K shell binding energy for K shell characteristic radiation to be produced.

C   If a vacancy from a recently ejected K shell electron is taken up by an M shell electron a photon of K_α radiation is emitted.

D   If a vacancy from a recently ejected K shell electron is taken up by an L shell electron a photon of K_α radiation is emitted.

E   Characteristic radiation emitted from outer shell electron transitions produce photons useful for diagnostic imaging.

Q6.6 CONCERNING BREMSSTRAHLUNG RADIATION PRODUCTION

A   It is distinctly different from continuous spectrum radiation production.

B   It is produced when a bombarding electron is deflected when passing close to the nucleus.

C   Most low energy Bremsstrahlung radiation produced below 20 kV is absorbed by the patient.

D   The production of Bremsstrahlung radiation below a certain kVp will cease.

E   Keeping all other parameters the same a reduction in the atomic number of the target will reduce the output of continuous radiation.

Q6.7 CONCERNING THE GENERAL DIAGNOSTIC X-RAY TUBE

A   More than 80% of the radiation emitted is characteristic radiation.

B   The anode does not rotate until a certain temperature is reached.

C   Virtually all of the emitted x-ray photons will have energy equivalent to the kVp of the tube.

D   Increasing the kVp moves the spectrum upwards and to the right.

E   Decreasing the mA narrows the spectrum and shifts it downwards.

Q6.8 THE X-RAY SPECTRUM MAY BE AFFECTED AS FOLLOWS

A   Decreasing the kVp moves the x-ray spectrum to the left and downwards.

B   A high frequency generator will produce more x-rays at higher energies compared to a full wave rectified generator.

C   Added filtration to the x-ray tube housing is designed to filter out higher energy photons.

D   If the anode target material is changed to that of a lower atomic number the characteristic radiation lines will shift to the right on the x-ray spectrum.

E   If the mA is increased the shape of the x-ray spectrum is unaltered.

Q6.9 CONCERNING THE X-RAY TUBE AND HOUSING

A   A high voltage potential is placed across the filament to produce electrons.

B   The positive cathode emits electrons by thermionic emission.

C   The rotating anode's bearings are lubricated with a synthetic oil.

D   The target rotates so as to distribute heat evenly over the disc.

E   The x-ray tube housing is designed to absorb any x-rays that escape from the tube other than those from the window.

Q6.10 THE FOLLOWING FEATURES OF THE ROTATING ANODE DISC ARE TRUE

A   It has a bevelled edge which the electron beam falls upon called the focal spot.

B   The actual focal spot size and effective focal spot size can be treated as equal for most x-ray tubes.

C   The most useful part of the x-ray beam produced at the focal spot lies perpendicular to the electron beam.

D   It may rotate at speeds of 3000 rpm or more.

E   Tungsten is the only target material used in diagnostic imaging equipment.

Q6.11 THE DOSE RECEIVED BY A PATIENT CAN BE MEASURED USING

A   Thermoluminescent dosimeters placed directly on the surface of the patient.

B   A Dose Area Product meter.

C   An ionisation chamber.

D   Thermoluminescent dosimeters placed directly on a standard phantom.

E   A star resolution grid.

Q6.12 THE FOLLOWING SHOULD BE RECORDED WHEN AN INDIVIDUAL IS EXPOSED TO A RADIOLOGICAL PROCEDURE

A Number of x-ray films.

B Focus to skin distance.

C The focal spot size.

D Type of examination.

E Screening times.

Q6.13 PATIENT RECORDS OF A RADIOLOGICAL EXPOSURE SHOULD INCLUDE

A The type of radionuclide administered.

B The exposure factors.

C The equipment used.

D The clinical evaluation of the image.

E A completed request form.

Q6.14 CONCERNING EXPOSURE RESTRICTION

A By selecting a lower kV the dose received by the patient is reduced.

B Lead filters of at least 2.5 mm are required to reduce the low energy component of the x-ray beam.

C The focus to skin distance should always be greater than 30 cm.

D Using image intensifier magnification can reduce the dose.

E Use of a grid reduces the dose.

Q6.15 METHODS TO REDUCE THE DOSE RECEIVED BY A PATIENT INCLUDES

A The use of automatic exposure controls (AEC).

B Minimising the number of CT slices.

C Collimation.

D The use of continuous screening in fluoroscopy.

E Making use of previous films.

Q6.16 THE FOLLOWING EQUIPMENT IS USED TO REDUCE PATIENT DOSE

A Fast screen-film combinations.

B Low attenuation materials for cassette fronts.

C Appropriate beam filtration.

D Anti-scatter grid.

E Pulsed fluoroscopy equipment.

Q6.17 THE FOLLOWING TECHNIQUES ARE USED TO REDUCE PATIENT DOSE

A The smallest focus to skin distance.

B The largest possible field size and good collimation.

C Compression of the patient where possible.

D Non-grid techniques.

E Collimation to exclude radiosensitive organs.

Answers

A6.1 CONCERNING THE PRODUCTION OF X-RAY PHOTONS FROM AN X-RAY TUBE

A False – The filament voltage is responsible for heating the filament so electrons can be emitted by thermionic emission (effectively boiled off).

B False – The electrons bombard the *positive* anode target.

C True.

D True.

E False – The tube has a vacuum otherwise the electrons would be scattered.

A6.2 ACCELERATED ELECTRONS IN AN X-RAY TUBE

A True – They need a lot of energy to bombard the anode and produce useful x-rays.

B False – The ratio is 100:1.

C True.

D True – The K shell binding energy of tungsten is 70 keV.

E False – The electrons cannot pass through glass. The insulated housing is in case an electrical fault occurs.

KEY CONCEPT

kV AND mA

- Peak tube voltage (kVp) = maximum potential difference across the tube and the highest possible photon energy.
- Tube current (mA) = equates to the number of accelerated electrons.

A6.3 CONCERNING HEAT REMOVAL FROM AN X-RAY TUBE

A   False – The molybdenum stem is highly insulative to prevent the transmission of excessive heat to the delicate bearings.

B   True – These systems are actively cooled.

C   False – It is surrounded by an oil bath.

D   True – The heat energy from the disc is radiated into the oil, then convected to the tube housing and finally to the open air.

E   True – The disc can store the energy temporarily and then release it to the oil by radiation. The anode can be called a temporary 'heat sink'.

A6.4 CONCERNING HIGH VOLTAGE GENERATORS

A   False – Self-rectifying voltage is an alternating voltage.

B   True.

C   True.

D   False – The full wave rectified generator will be at the peak kVp for double the time than the self-rectifying generator.

E   True.

A6.5 CONCERNING CHARACTERISTIC RADIATION

A   False – Electrons ejected from the valence shells will not have any outer shell electrons to take their place and thus cannot emit characteristic radiation.

B   True.

C   False – A $K\beta$ photon will be produced, with the energy equal to the difference of binding energies between the K and M shell.

D   True – The production of an x-ray photon from the transition from the next adjacent shell into the K shell is called K_α radiation.

E   False – The energy of these photons is low.

> ### KEY CONCEPT
> ### X-RAY PRODUCTION
>
> There are two processes by which x-rays are produced.
> - **Bremsstrahlung (continuous) radiation:** Is created when an accelerated electron passes very close to (even closer than the orbiting K shell electrons) and is deflected by the nucleus. It is slowed and loses energy. This energy is converted into a single x-ray photon.
> - **Characteristic radiation:** Is created when an accelerated electron strikes and removes an orbiting electron in any shell except the valence shell. The energy of the incident electron must be greater than the binding energy of the orbiting electron to remove it. Once the electron has been removed there is a vacancy within the shell which is filled by an electron from an outer shell. This transition releases an x-ray photon with an energy equal to the difference between the binding energies of the removed electron and the replacing electron. Photon energy will be greater when electrons are removed from shells closer to the nucleus as their binding energies will be greater.

A6.6 CONCERNING BREMSSTRAHLUNG RADIATION PRODUCTION

A False – Continuous spectrum radiation and Bremsstrahlung radiation are the same phenomenon.

B True.

C False – The tube and its window absorb virtually all of these low energy photons.

D False – Bremsstrahlung will always be produced.

E True.

A6.7 CONCERNING THE GENERAL DIAGNOSTIC X-RAY TUBE

A False – More than 80% of the radiation is Bremsstrahlung radiation.

B False – The anode rotates every time the tube is energised. Only dental x-ray units have stationary anodes.

C   False – The average energy of an x-ray spectrum (also known as the effective energy) is around 30% to 50% of the kVp.

D   True.

E   False – mA is responsible for the quantity of the photons and not the energy.

A6.8 THE X-RAY SPECTRUM MAY BE AFFECTED AS FOLLOWS

A   True.

B   True.

C   False – It is the low energy photons that are filtered.

D   False – An atom with a lower atomic number will have a lower K shell electron binding energy.

E   True.

A6.9 CONCERNING THE X-RAY TUBE AND HOUSING

A   False – Only a small voltage (around 10 V) is needed to make the filament glow.

B   False – The cathode is negative.

C   False – They are lubricated with solid silver.

D   True.

E   True – This reduces scatter and additional dose to the patient and operator.

A6.10 THE FOLLOWING FEATURES OF THE ROTATING ANODE DISC ARE TRUE

A   True.

B   False.

C   True.

D   True.

E   False – Other materials such as molybdenum are used.

X-RAY SPECTRUM, QUALITY AND QUANTITY

The x-ray spectrum graph of a typical x-ray tube depicts the tube voltage along the x-axis and the number of photons on the y-axis. The graph displays a hump then peaks. The hump represents Bremsstrahlung radiation (continuous radiation) and the peaks represent characteristic radiation. The graph finishes and meets the x-axis at the maximum kVp applied across the tube. Increasing the kVp increases the maximum possible energy a photon could have and increases the average energy of the x-ray spectrum thus the curve is shifted upwards and to the right. Decreasing the kVp does the opposite to the curve.

Beam quality describes the energy range of radiation available (or spectrum). It is dependent on the kVp. It is **independent of mAs**, therefore changing the mAs will not change the shape of the spectrum.

Beam intensity or quantity describes the amount of radiation within the beam (number of photons per unit area per period of time). It is dependent on the mAs across the tube and the kV.

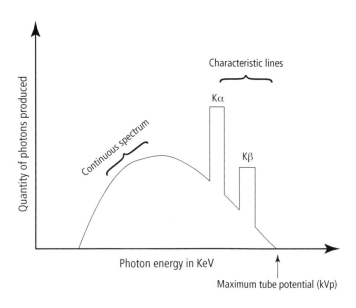

FIGURE 6.1 A typical x-ray spectrum

KEY CONCEPT

EFFECTIVE AND ACTUAL FOCAL SPOT SIZE

The actual focal spot is bigger than the effective focal spot due to the electron beam being projected onto a bevelled edge. The larger actual focal spot size allows heat to be dissipated more evenly.

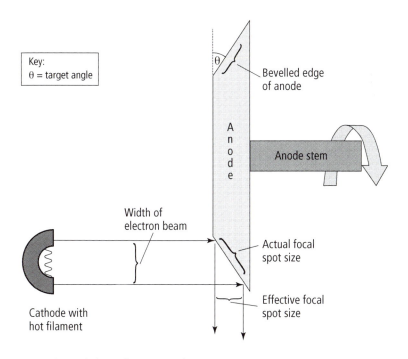

FIGURE 6.2 Lateral view of an x-ray tube

A6.11 THE DOSE RECEIVED BY A PATIENT CAN BE MEASURED USING

A True.

B True.

C True – This can measure air kerma rate at a given distance from the tube and an estimate of the patient entrance surface dose can be made from known exposure factors.

D True.

E False – This is used to measure the focal spot size.

A6.12 THE FOLLOWING SHOULD BE RECORDED WHEN AN INDIVIDUAL IS EXPOSED TO A RADIOLOGICAL PROCEDURE

A True.

B True.

C False – This is measured during the quality assurance programme.

D True.

E True.

A6.13 PATIENT RECORDS OF A RADIOLOGICAL EXPOSURE SHOULD INCLUDE

A True.

B True.

C True.

D True.

E True.

A6.14 CONCERNING EXPOSURE RESTRICTION

A False – By using a higher kV the patient dose is reduced.

B False – Aluminium filters of at least 2.5 mm should be used to reduce the low energy component of the x-ray beam.

C True – The focus to skin distance should never be less than 30 cm.

D False – Magnifying images increases the dose.

E False – Grids increase the dose.

A6.15 METHODS TO REDUCE THE DOSE RECEIVED BY A PATIENT INCLUDES

A True.

B True.

C True.

D False – Use pulsed screening which will reduce the screening time and hence the dose.

E True – Further studies may not be required if the information is on previous images.

A6.16 THE FOLLOWING EQUIPMENT IS USED TO REDUCE PATIENT DOSE

A True.

B True.

C True.

D False – This increases patient dose.

E True.

A6.17 THE FOLLOWING TECHNIQUES ARE USED TO REDUCE PATIENT DOSE

A False – The largest practicable skin to focus distance should be used, never less than 30 cm.

B False – Use the smallest field size and good collimation.

C True.

D True.

E True.

CHAPTER 7

General principles of radiology

Q7.1 CONCERNING IMAGE UNSHARPNESS

A   Decreasing grain size results in a reduction of image unsharpness.

B   Increasing film to focus distance results in a reduction of image unsharpness.

C   Decreasing object to focus distance results in reduced image unsharpness.

D   Reducing focal spot size reduces image unsharpness.

E   Increasing the target angle reduces image unsharpness.

Q7.2 CONCERNING LINEAR TOMOGRAPHY

A It is a useful technique to image a particular plane within the patient.

B The level of pivot is not important when choosing the slice level of the patient.

C The tomographic angle controls the thickness of cut.

D The dose tends to be greater than for conventional radiography.

E Zoneography requires a greater angle of pivot compared to linear tomography.

Q7.3 THE FOLLOWING ARE TRUE OF GEOMETRICAL UNSHARPNESS

A A typical overcouch tube delivers an ideal point source of x-rays.

B The greater the focal spot size the greater the geometrical unsharpness.

C Reducing the object–film distance will reduce geometrical unsharpness.

D Patient movement will increase geometrical unsharpness.

E Can be reduced by using a shorter exposure time.

Q7.4 THE FOLLOWING FACTORS AFFECT GEOMETRICAL UNSHARPNESS

A Patient movement.

B Film to focus distance.

C Tapering thickness of the thoracic aorta.

D Focal spot size.

E Film grain size.

Q7.5 THE FOLLOWING FACTORS AFFECT MOVEMENT UNSHARPNESS

A Exposure time.

B Use of an intensifying screen.

C Focal spot size.

D Patient immobilisation.

E Film grain size.

Q7.6 THE FOLLOWING ARE TRUE OF INTENSIFYING SCREENS

A They improve resolution.

B They improve unsharpness.

C They reduce patient dose.

D They reduce the loading on x-ray equipment.

E They are used in all plain film radiography.

Q7.7 CONCERNING INTENSIFICATION SCREENS

A Light produced by the intensifying screen only contributes to 50% of the image.

B The intensification factor of a screen is the ratio of the x-ray exposure required without screens over the exposure required with screens.

C The intensification factor is related to screen speed.

D Contact between the screen and film is not of importance.

E Calcium tungstate screens are faster than rare earth screens.

Q7.8 THE FOLLOWING ARE TRUE OF RARE EARTH SCREENS

A Maximum speed is reached using a tube potential of around 80 kVp.

B They convert x-ray photons into light photons via the photoelectric effect.

C Terbium activated lanthanum oxybromide screens produce blue light.

D Terbium activated gadolinium oxysulphide screens produce red light.

E They can have a thinner coating of phosphor and produce the same intensification compared to calcium tungstate screens.

Q7.9 SCREEN SPEED IS AFFECTED BY THE FOLLOWING

A Temperature.

B Thickness.

C Backing material.

D kVp.

E Size of intensification compound crystals.

Q7.10 THE FOLLOWING FACTORS ARE DIRECTLY INVOLVED IN IMAGE QUALITY

A Unsharpness.

B Contrast.

C Artefact.

D   Age of patient.

E   Noise.

Q7.11 THE FOLLOWING ARE TRUE OF CONTRAST

A   It is the ability to see two different densities of grey on a plain film.

B   It is the ability to see two different lines close together on a film of the same optical density.

C   Contrast in a plain film image is due to differences in tissue attenuation of x-rays.

D   Contrast agents always increase the attenuation of x-rays.

E   The greater the difference in attenuation coefficient of adjacent structures the greater the contrast.

Q7.12 THE FOLLOWING ARE TRUE OF A BEAM OF X-RAYS EMERGING FROM A PATIENT

A   It contains unattenuated radiation.

B   Differences in attenuation of the primary beam within the patient will produce image contrast.

C   It continues to diverge.

D   It will not contain scattered radiation.

E   The beam will be 'softened'.

Q7.13 CONCERNING SUBJECT CONTRAST

A If the thickness of a structure increases the contrast will increase.

B It is dependent on how close the adjacent structures are together.

C It is not affected by the difference of linear attenuation coefficients (LAC) of two adjacent structures.

D It is affected by the difference in density between two adjacent structures.

E It is not affected by the difference in atomic number of two adjacent structures.

Q7.14 THE FOLLOWING WILL INCREASE THE NOISE IN AN IMAGE

A Use of intensifying screens.

B Use of a rare earth intensifying screen compared to a calcium tungstate screen.

C Increasing the kV and keeping all other parameters the same.

D Increasing the mAs and keeping all other parameters the same.

E Using a low dose technique.

Q7.15 THE SIGNAL TO NOISE RATIO (SNR) IS INCREASED IN THE FOLLOWING INSTANCES

A Use of double intensifying screens.

B Using a 'fast' film.

C Using a lower kV and increasing mAs.

D   Using a lower mAs and increasing kV.

E   Using a thicker layer of phosphor in the intensifying screen.

Q7.16 THE FOLLOWING TECHNIQUES TYPICALLY DO NOT USE GRIDS

A   Mammography.

B   Paediatric radiography.

C   Radiography of digits.

D   Abdominal radiography.

E   Pelvic radiography.

Q7.17 THE FOLLOWING ARE TRUE OF THE ANTI-SCATTER GRID

A   Focused grids can only be used in one orientation.

B   They reduce patient dose.

C   They remove all scatter.

D   Unfocused grids can be used with any focus–film distance (FFD).

E   The filtering components that form the grid are typically made from heavy metals such as lead.

Q7.18 A TYPICAL ANTI-SCATTER GRID WILL REDUCE THE FOLLOWING

A Scatter reaching the film.

B Primary beam radiation reaching the film.

C Patient dose.

D Contrast.

E Film speed.

Q7.19 THE FOLLOWING ARE TRUE OF FOCAL SPOT SIZE

A Effective focal spot size is usually greater than actual focal spot size.

B Effective focal spot size can be measured using a 'star test' device.

C Effective focal spot size can be measured using a 'pinhole' device.

D If the target angle decreases the size of the effective focal spot increases.

E If the focal spot size decreases so will the resolution.

Q7.20 THE FOLLOWING WILL REDUCE SCATTER REACHING THE FILM

A Patient compression.

B Use of a grid.

C Increasing the kV.

D Reducing focal spot size.

E Size of field exposed.

Q7.21 THE FOLLOWING ARE TRUE OF BEAM FILTRATION AFTER PASSING THROUGH A COPPER FILTER

A The beam will be softened.

B Mean energy increases.

C Beam intensity decreases.

D Beam filtration increases patient dose.

E Reduces the maximum photon energy of the beam.

Q7.22 THE FOLLOWING ARE USEFUL PROPERTIES OF FILTERS

A Removal of low energy photons.

B They increase the intensity of the beam.

C They reduce the half value layer of the beam.

D The main purpose of the second filtration layer of a compound filter is to remove more of the lower energy photons from the unfiltered primary beam.

E They supplement inherent filtration of the x-ray tube itself.

Q7.23 THE FOLLOWING ARE TRUE OF SCATTER

A Using an air gap reduces the amount of scatter reaching the image receptor.

B Scatter is reduced by increasing the field size.

C Scatter produced at diagnostic energies is predominantly in the forward direction.

D Scatter reduces contrast in the image.

E The ratio of scatter to primary beam can be as high as 10:1.

Q7.24 EXTRA FOCAL RADIATION

A Contributes to patient dose.

B Contributes to scatter in the image.

C Can be caused by stray electrons emitted from the cathode striking the anode outside the focal spot.

D Is mostly removed by the tube housing and added filtration.

E Does not affect unsharpness.

Q7.25 CONCERNING THE AIR GAP TECHNIQUE

A It reduces scatter reaching the image receptor.

B It is typically used in conjunction with a grid.

C It results in image magnification.

D It reduces contrast.

E It is more effective with smaller gaps.

Q7.26 REGARDING THE GAMMA OF A FILM–SCREEN COMBINATION

A It is dependent on film crystal size.

B A high gamma film gives greater contrast over a narrower range of photon energy.

C It can be calculated from the gradient of the characteristic curve of a film.

D It is independent of the screen material used.

E Small crystals in the film will require less relative energy to form a latent image compared to larger crystals.

Q7.27 CONCERNING THE CHARACTERISTIC CURVE OF A FILM

A Is a plot of film optical density against log relative exposure.

B The gamma of a film–screen combination can be calculated from the curve.

C The latitude describes the desired range of relative energies that will produce an image in the useful optical density range.

D It is constant at all times.

E An unexposed but developed film will have an optical density of zero.

Q7.28 CONCERNING CHANGES IN FILM DEVELOPING CONDITIONS

A Reducing developer temperature reduces fog.

B Developer is stored at minus five degrees or below.

C Film gamma is constant and is not affected by development conditions.

D Changes in the concentration of developer does not alter the speed.

E Changes in developing time does not alter the film gamma.

Answers

A7.1 CONCERNING IMAGE UNSHARPNESS

A True.

B True.

C False.

D True.

E False – Increasing the target angle leads to an increase in the effective focal spot size and hence increased image unsharpness.

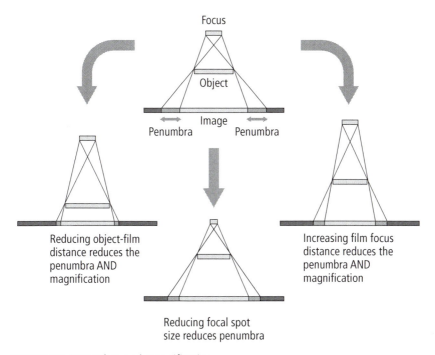

FIGURE 7.1 Penumbra and magnification

A7.2 CONCERNING LINEAR TOMOGRAPHY

A True.

B False – The level of pivot is the level at which the beam will be relatively still and create a sharp image of the structures.

C True.

D True.

E False – Zoneography is similar to linear tomography but uses a smaller angle of pivot, such as 5–10 degrees.

A7.3 THE FOLLOWING ARE TRUE OF GEOMETRICAL UNSHARPNESS

A False – No tube will deliver a true ideal point source, the focal spot will always have area.

B True – The penumbra will be greater.

C True – There is less distance for the penumbra to expand and increase the unsharpness.

D False – Patient movement results in movement unsharpness.

E False.

A7.4 THE FOLLOWING FACTORS AFFECT GEOMETRICAL UNSHARPNESS

A False – This is movement unsharpness.

B True.

C False – This is an example of absorption unsharpness.

D True.

E False – This results in image unsharpness.

A7.5 THE FOLLOWING FACTORS AFFECT MOVEMENT UNSHARPNESS

A True.

B True.

C False.

D True.

E False.

KEY CONCEPT
IMAGE UNSHARPNESS

Geometrical unsharpness is affected by:
- film-focus distance
- object-film distance
- focal spot size.

Movement unsharpness is affected by:
- patient movement
- exposure time.

Absorption unsharpness is affected by:
- gradual change in thickness of an object being imaged, e.g. the edge of a blood vessel.

A7.6 THE FOLLOWING ARE TRUE OF INTENSIFYING SCREENS

A False – The light photons produced in the screen diverge from their point of production, blurring the image and reducing resolution.

B False – As above.

C True – The intensifying screen converts a single x-ray photon into many light photons which form the image, reducing the exposure required.

D True.

E False – Due to the blurring nature of intensification screens they are not suitable for all plain radiography such as extremities.

A7.7 CONCERNING INTENSIFICATION SCREENS

A False – The light produced by the intensification screen contributes to around 90% of the image.

B True.

C True.

D False – Poor screen–film contact contributes to blurring of the image.

E False – Rare earth screens are more efficient than calcium tungstate.

A7.8 THE FOLLOWING ARE TRUE OF RARE EARTH SCREENS

A True – Above and below 80 kVp the screen speeds decrease.

B True.

C True.

D False – Green light is produced; x-ray film is not very sensitive to red light which is why the safe light in a dark room is red.

E True – As rare earth screens are more efficient the thickness of the phosphor layer can be reduced.

A7.9 SCREEN SPEED IS AFFECTED BY THE FOLLOWING

A True – Screen speed increases the cooler the screen temperature is.

B True – Thicker screens capture more x-ray photons and more light photons are produced.

C True – The more light reflective the backing material the more light is reflected back towards the film.

D True – Rare earth screens have a peak phosphorescence at around 80 kVp.

E True – The larger the crystal the greater the chance of it photoelectrically absorbing an x-ray photon.

A7.10 THE FOLLOWING FACTORS ARE DIRECTLY INVOLVED IN IMAGE QUALITY

A True.

B True.

C True.

D False.

E True.

A7.11 THE FOLLOWING ARE TRUE OF CONTRAST

A True.

B False – This is the resolution.

C True.

D False – Both positive (substances with high x-ray attenuation, e.g. barium in the GI tract) and negative (substances with low x-ray attenuation, e.g. air in CT colonography) contrast agents can be used.

E True.

A7.12 THE FOLLOWING ARE TRUE OF A BEAM OF X-RAYS EMERGING FROM A PATIENT

A True.

B True.

C True.

D False.

E False – The beam will have been 'filtered' by the patient so will become 'harder'.

A7.13 CONCERNING SUBJECT CONTRAST

A True.

B False – This is resolution.

C False.

D True.

E False.

A7.14 THE FOLLOWING WILL INCREASE THE NOISE IN AN IMAGE

A True.

B True.

C True.

D False.

E True.

KEY CONCEPT

FACTORS INFLUENCING NOISE AND SNR

- **Noise:** Is the representation of the fluctuating number of photons absorbed in the input screen due to the statistical variation of photons per unit area.
- **Signal to noise ratio (SNR):** Is the ratio of the true signal (i.e. the photons actually forming the image) to the amount of unwanted noise.

$$\downarrow photons => \uparrow noise => \downarrow SNR$$
$$\uparrow photons => \downarrow noise => \uparrow SNR$$

A7.15 THE SIGNAL TO NOISE RATIO (SNR) IS INCREASED IN THE FOLLOWING INSTANCES

A False – The SNR is reduced as fewer photons form the image and therefore noise is increased.

B False – The SNR is reduced as fewer photons are used to produce the image.

C True – More photons will form the image, therefore the SNR is increased.

D False – Fewer photons will form the image and the SNR will decrease.

E False – The screen will be faster as more photons will be captured and converted into light photons.

A7.16 THE FOLLOWING TECHNIQUES TYPICALLY DO NOT USE GRIDS

A False.

B True.

C True – Negligible scatter is produced by extremities.

D False.

E False.

A7.17 THE FOLLOWING ARE TRUE OF THE ANTI-SCATTER GRID

A True.

B False – Grids increase patient dose.

C False – Scattered radiation travelling parallel to the primary beam will pass through the grid.

D False – Eventually, as the FFD increases grid 'cut-off' will occur.

E True.

A7.18 A TYPICAL ANTI-SCATTER GRID WILL REDUCE THE FOLLOWING

A True.

B True – The grid will inevitably filter out some of the primary beam.

C False.

D False – Removing scatter will improve contrast.

E False – The grid has nothing to do with film speed.

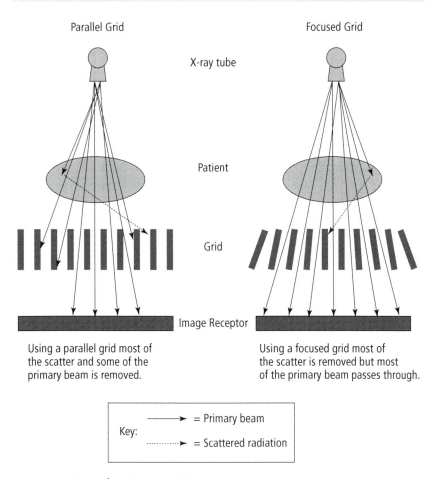

FIGURE 7.2 Types of anti-scatter grid

A7.19 THE FOLLOWING ARE TRUE OF FOCAL SPOT SIZE

A False.

B True.

C True.

D False – A reduction in target angle will reduce the effective focal spot size.

E False – The smaller the focal spot the less penumbra or edge blurring that will occur when it passes a structure.

A7.20 THE FOLLOWING WILL REDUCE SCATTER REACHING THE FILM

A True – This reduces the volume of tissue in which scattering processes can occur.

B True.

C False – This increases the energy of scattered radiation, therefore more reaches the film.

D False – Focal spot size is independent of scatter production.

E True – The smaller the field the less volume scattering events can occur within.

A7.21 THE FOLLOWING ARE TRUE OF BEAM FILTRATION AFTER PASSING THROUGH A COPPER FILTER

A False – It will be hardened as more of the lower energy photons will have been filtered out.

B True – Mean energy will increase as lower energy photons will have been removed from the beam.

C True – Fewer photons will pass per unit area per unit time as the lower energy photons will have been filtered out.

D False – The lower energy photons are filtered out, therefore reducing patient dose.

E False – The maximum photon energy stays the same as the high energy photons can still pass through the filter.

A7.22 THE FOLLOWING ARE USEFUL PROPERTIES OF FILTERS

A True.

B False – Beam filtration reduces the intensity of the beam.

C False – Filtration increases the half value layer of the beam as the filtered beam is more penetrating.

D False – The second layer removes any characteristic photons produced by first filter.

E True – The x-ray tube itself removes the lowest energy photons from the beam and then filters remove more.

A7.23 THE FOLLOWING ARE TRUE OF SCATTER

A   True – A proportion of scatter that would have otherwise reached the image receptor now misses it as it is further away.

B   False – Reducing the field size decreases the volume within which scattering events can occur.

C   True.

D   True.

E   True.

A7.24 EXTRA FOCAL RADIATION

A   True – Any radiation reaching the patient contributes to dose.

B   True.

C   True.

D   True.

E   False – Extra focal radiation effectively produces a large subtle penumbra of its own, increasing geometric unsharpness.

A7.25 CONCERNING THE AIR GAP TECHNIQUE

A   True.

B   False – The air gap is used as an alternative to the grid.

C   True – The beam continues to diverge, therefore the image will be magnified.

D   False – Its purpose is to increase contrast by reducing scatter.

E   False – It is more effective with larger gaps.

A7.26 REGARDING THE GAMMA OF A FILM–SCREEN COMBINATION

A   False – It is dependent on the range of crystal sizes.

B   True.

C   True – This is the definition of film gamma.

D   False – Altering the screen material will alter the gamma.

E   False – The larger crystals need less relative energy to form latent images on the film.

A7.27 CONCERNING THE CHARACTERISTIC CURVE OF A FILM

A True.

B True.

C True.

D False – The characteristic curve of a film can be affected by developing conditions.

E False – The film will always have a baseline optical density or fog level.

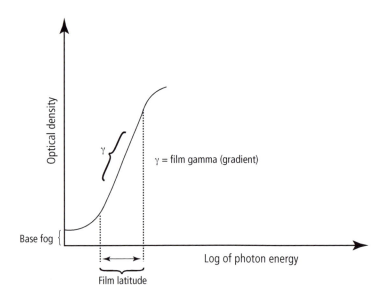

FIGURE 7.3 A typical film characteristic curve

A7.28 CONCERNING CHANGES IN FILM DEVELOPING CONDITIONS

A True.

B False – It can be stored at room temperature.

C False – Gamma increases initially with an increase in developer temperature but then drops as the degree of fog increases.

D False – Any change in developing conditions will alter the film speed, fog level, gamma and contrast.

E False – As above.

CHAPTER 8

Computed and digital radiography

Q8.1 CONCERNING COMPUTED RADIOGRAPHY

A   The film in the cassette is replaced by a photostimulable phosphor plate.

B   Electrons are promoted from a conduction band into a valence band.

C   Electrons can decay into energy traps after promotion.

D   Laser light can give trapped electrons enough energy to leave energy traps.

E   Photostimulable plates used in plain radiography are cheap and of single use.

Q8.2 REGARDING THE IMAGE STORED ON A PHOTOSTIMULABLE PHOSPHOR PLATE (PSP)

A The image can be read by passing a laser beam across an exposed plate.

B Developer concentration affects the speed at which the plate is read.

C The latent image is stable so plate reading can take place a long while after the image is taken.

D The light photons released by trapped electrons returning to their valence band are all of a certain wavelength.

E Image artefacts due to PSP faults are incredibly rare.

Q8.3 REGARDING IMAGE PRODUCTION FROM A PHOTOSTIMULABLE PHOSPHOR PLATE

A The latent image stored on the plate can decay if not read promptly.

B Resolution is affected by the thickness of the photostimulable phosphor layer.

C Latitude is fixed.

D The relative exposure vs. output signal plot is a straight line.

E Slow read speed does not affect image quality.

Q8.4 REGARDING DIGITAL RADIOGRAPHY

A The charge coupled device converts photons into an electronic signal.

B The input phosphor is coupled to the charge coupled device (CCD) by fibre optics.

C   Both flat panel array detectors and charge coupled devices have dead areas.

D   Resolution on a flat panel array is limited to the width of the detector elements.

E   Image latitude can be altered after the image has been taken.

Q8.5 THE FOLLOWING ARE TRUE OF ANALOGUE IMAGES

A   The image is made up of numerous screen pixels.

B   Can easily be stored directly on a computer.

C   It is created by a beam of varying electron intensity scanning across a phosphor screen.

D   Can be recorded onto a magnetic tape.

E   Is used in CT.

Q8.6 THE FOLLOWING ARE TRUE OF DIGITAL IMAGES

A   The digital image is made up of pixels.

B   Each pixel is given a binary number which gives its greyscale level.

C   Each pixel is given a binary number which gives its point on the screen.

D   The digital image can be directly displayed on a cathode ray monitor.

E   Digital information can be modified by a computer.

Q8.7 THE FOLLOWING MANIPULATIONS OF DIGITAL IMAGES CAN BE UNDERTAKEN

A   Windowing.

B   Edge enhancement.

C   Frame averaging.

D   Vignetting.

E   Background subtraction.

Q8.8 THE FOLLOWING IMAGING MODALITIES TYPICALLY PROCESS IMAGES DIGITALLY

A   CT.

B   Mammography.

C   Gamma cameras.

D   Spiral CT.

E   Positron emission tomography.

Q8.9 THE FOLLOWING ARE TRUE OF DIGITAL SUBTRACTION ANGIOGRAPHY (DSA)

A   It requires no contrast agent to be administered to the patient.

B   It requires a mask image to be taken before subtraction can occur.

C   Quantum noise is greater in the digitally subtracted image.

D Requires a higher mA compared to normal screening.

E Movement of the patient or organ does not affect the final image.

Q8.10 CONTRAST AGENTS USED IN DIGITAL SUBTRACTION ANGIOGRAPHY (DSA)

A Are typically iodine based.

B Are stable and non-toxic.

C Are made from high viscosity materials.

D Are made of a material which has low x-ray absorption.

E Are easily excreted.

Q8.11 IN DIGITAL SUBTRACTION ANGIOGRAPHY MISREGISTRATION (WHERE STRUCTURES IN THE MASK IMAGE AND CONTRAST IMAGE ARE NOT IN EXACTLY THE SAME PLACE)

A Can occur from cardiac motion.

B Can occur from peristalsis.

C Can be caused by x-ray signal instability.

D Can produce artefacts.

E Can be resolved by moving the mask image.

Q8.12 THE FOLLOWING ARE TRUE OF A CATHODE RAY DISPLAY MONITOR

A It contains an anode and a cathode.

B Contains a phosphor coated cathode.

C The electron beam can be deflected.

D The voltage applied between the electron gun and phosphor screen is always constant.

E Cathode ray monitors contain thin film transistor (TFT) display screens.

Answers

A8.1 CONCERNING COMPUTED RADIOGRAPHY

A True.

B False – The electrons are promoted from the valence band into the conduction band by the absorption of photons.

C True.

D True – This is how the phosphor plate is read with a laser beam scanning to and fro across the plate.

E False – The plates are expensive but can be reused.

A8.2 REGARDING THE IMAGE STORED ON A PHOTOSTIMULABLE PHOSPHOR PLATE (PSP)

A True.

B False – No chemicals are used in this process.

C False – The trapped electrons will slowly over time return to their valence band resulting in image quality degradation.

D True.

E False – Eventually every PSP will have to be replaced as they become worn or scratched.

A8.3 REGARDING IMAGE PRODUCTION FROM A PHOTOSTIMULABLE PHOSPHOR PLATE

A True.

B True – A thicker phosphor layer causes more scatter, therefore reducing resolution.

C False – The latitude can be altered to a certain degree to provide the best quality image.

D True – Image parameters such as latitude can be altered during post processing.

E False – Read speed should be quick to ensure as much of the emitted light photons are detected.

A8.4 REGARDING DIGITAL RADIOGRAPHY

A True.

B True – The input phosphor is coupled to the CCD by fibre optics to increase efficiency.

C True.

D True.

E True.

A8.5 THE FOLLOWING ARE TRUE OF ANALOGUE IMAGES

A False.

B False.

C True.

D True.

E False.

A8.6 THE FOLLOWING ARE TRUE OF DIGITAL IMAGES

A True.

B True.

C True.

D False – It needs to be converted by a digital-analogue converter.

E True.

KEY CONCEPT

ANALOGUE VS. DIGITAL IMAGING

An analogue image, as displayed on a cathode ray monitor, is created by a beam of varying electron intensity scanning across a phosphor screen. This causes the phosphor coating to fluoresce at different intensities, thus creating an image. This can be converted into a digital image by an analogue-digital converter.

A digital image is made up of pixels. Each pixel represents a greyscale level and a location within the image grid.

Modifications such as windowing, enhancing and image manipulation are possible with digital images.

A8.7 THE FOLLOWING MANIPULATIONS OF DIGITAL IMAGES CAN BE UNDERTAKEN

A True – This is selection of a certain level of greyscale which allows better interpretation of information.

B True – Edges on images can be enhanced by computer.

C True.

D False – Vignetting is the phenomenon of losing light photons at the edge of an image while passing through an image intensifier.

E True – The same value is subtracted from all pixels; this increases contrast.

A8.8 THE FOLLOWING IMAGING MODALITIES TYPICALLY PROCESS IMAGES DIGITALLY

A True.

B False – Most mammography departments typically use plain film.

C True.

D True.

E True.

A8.9 THE FOLLOWING ARE TRUE OF DIGITAL SUBTRACTION ANGIOGRAPHY (DSA)

A False.

B True.

C True – The signal to noise ratio increases.

D True – This is to reduce the noise in the subtracted image to an acceptable level.

E False – This will introduce unsharpness.

KEY CONCEPT

DIGITAL SUBTRACTION ANGIOGRAPHY (DSA)

A background image is taken and stored before contrast is introduced (mask image). Contrast is introduced into the vessel of interest and a further image is taken (contrast image). The first image is subtracted from the second. Therefore all the background information will be removed and the contrast filled vessel will remain (subtracted image).

A8.10 CONTRAST AGENTS USED IN DIGITAL SUBTRACTION ANGIOGRAPHY (DSA)

A True.

B True.

C False – They are made of a material which has a low viscosity.

D False – They are made of a material which has a high x-ray absorption.

E True.

A8.11 IN DIGITAL SUBTRACTION ANGIOGRAPHY MISREGISTRATION (WHERE STRUCTURES IN THE MASK IMAGE AND CONTRAST IMAGE ARE NOT IN EXACTLY THE SAME PLACE)

A True – Misregistration can occur from both patient and tissue movement.

B True.

C True.

D True.

E True.

A8.12 THE FOLLOWING ARE TRUE OF A CATHODE RAY DISPLAY MONITOR

A True.

B False – The phosphor screen is the anode.

C True.

D False.

E False – TFT screens contain no cathode ray tubes. TFTs are the basis of flat screen technology.

KEY CONCEPT

THE CATHODE RAY DISPLAY MONITOR

Within the cathode ray monitor electrons are accelerated from a negative cathode in a fine beam and strike the phosphor coated anode screen. As the beam scans across the anode it causes the phosphor to glow, producing an image. The applied voltage varies depending on the desired brightness. This produces contrast in the image.

CHAPTER 9

Computed tomography

Q9.1 THE FOLLOWING FACTORS AFFECT THE SPATIAL RESOLUTION OF CT

A Pitch.

B Slice width.

C Pixel size.

D Window range.

E Focal spot size.

Q9.2 CONCERNING SPATIAL RESOLUTION OF THE CT SCANNER

A Noise affects spatial resolution.

B Volume averaging does not affect spatial resolution.

C It can be tested using a Perspex phantom containing progressively reducing diameter holes filled with water.

D Is improved by reducing detector element size.

E Modern CT scanners are so fast at image acquisition patient movement produces negligible reduction in spatial resolution.

Q9.3 THE FOLLOWING ARE TRUE OF CONTRAST IN CT IMAGING

A Contrast can be defined as the difference in attenuation between structures, therefore allowing distinction between them.

B An example of positive contrast is insufflation of air into the rectum.

C An example of negative contrast agent is the injection of an iodinated contrast agent intravenously.

D Noise reduces contrast.

E Reducing slice thickness reduces contrast.

Q9.4 CONCERNING CT SCANNER COMPONENTS

A Tube loading is lower compared with plain radiography due to tube rotation.

B Collimation of the beam occurs before passing through the patient.

C   The anode–cathode axis of the CT x-ray tube is perpendicular to the fan beam.

D   Collimation is fixed.

E   A typical kV applied across the CT tube is 120 kV.

Q9.5 THE FOLLOWING FACTORS ARE MEASURED DURING A CT SCAN

A   The detector measures transmitted x-ray intensity.

B   X-ray beam attenuation.

C   Linear attenuation coefficient of tissue.

D   Patient weight.

E   Effective dose.

Q9.6 THE FOLLOWING FACTORS ARE USED TO CALCULATE DOSE LENGTH PRODUCT IN CT

A   CT dose index.

B   Slice thickness.

C   Tube current.

D   Patient weight.

E   Region being imaged.

Q9.7 THE FOLLOWING CT MEASUREMENTS MATCH THEIR UNITS

A CT dose index is measured in mGy.cm.

B Dose length product is measured in mGy.

C Tube potential difference is measured in kV.

D Tube current is measured in milliamps (mA).

E CT number is measured in Hounsfield units (HU).

Q9.8 CONCERNING THE VOXEL IN CT IMAGING

A Voxel is an abbreviation for 'volume element'.

B It represents a definable region within a CT slice matrix.

C It is displayed in a three-dimensional fashion on an image display.

D It is a three-dimensional region within the scan slice matrix.

E A voxel is displayed as a pixel on a display monitor.

Q9.9 THE FOLLOWING METHODS CAN BE USED FOR IMAGE PRODUCTION IN CT

A Simple back projection.

B Digital subtraction.

C Fourier transformation.

D Filtered back projection.

E Use of a pulse height analyser.

Q9.10 REGARDING CT IMAGE ARTEFACTS

A A hip replacement would give rise to a streak artefact.

B Motion artefacts are caused by voxels being occupied by different parts of a moving structure at different times.

C Detector malfunction produces ring artefacts.

D Platinum cerebral aneurysm coils produce star artefacts.

E A faulty CT scanner table that moves abnormally during a scan will produce star artefacts.

Q9.11 THE FOLLOWING ARE CAUSES OF ARTEFACT IN CT SCAN IMAGES

A Aliasing artefact.

B Geometrical artefact.

C Beam hardening.

D Tube heat rating.

E Ring artefact.

Q9.12 THE FOLLOWING ARE TRUE OF DETECTORS USED IN CT

A Gas filled ionisation detectors are more efficient than solid state detectors.

B Sodium iodide detectors have less afterglow compared to bismuth germinate.

C Xenon gas can be used to fill ionisation chamber detectors.

D Signal from adjacent detectors can be coupled together to increase slice thickness.

E Gas filled ionisation chambers operate at normal atmospheric pressure.

Q9.13 THE FOLLOWING ARE TRUE OF DOSE IN CT IMAGING

A Reducing slice thickness reduces patient dose.

B Noise reduction often leads to an increased patient dose.

C An obese patient requires increased dose to produce an image with an acceptable noise level.

D Good quality control is necessary to ensure patient dose is as low as possible.

E A high resolution CT chest will deliver greater dose per slice than a routine chest CT.

Q9.14 REGARDING CT DOSIMETRY

A The CTDI is the integral of the dose along the axis of the patient from a single slice multiplied by the nominal thickness of the slice.

B Weighted CTDI takes into account the spatial distribution of dose within the patient in the scan plane

C $CTDI_w$ is measured in mSv.

D CTDI is related to the absorbed dose.

E Organ doses from a CT examination can be calculated by dividing the CDTI by the appropriate conversion factor.

Q9.15 CONCERNING CT DOSES, THE FOLLOWING ARE TRUE

A CT dose is proportional to the x-ray tube current (mA).

B CT dose is proportional to the gantry rotation time.

C CT dose is proportional to the pitch.

D CT dose is proportional to the mAs divided by the pitch.

E CT dose decreases as the kVp is increased.

Q9.16 REGARDING CT

A Under IRR 99 diagnostic reference levels for all examinations are required to compare local doses against a standard.

B UK Diagnostic Reference Levels for CT are given in terms of CTDI and DLP.

C For similar image quality multi-slice scanners are lower dose than single slice scanners.

D The effective dose in CT can be calculated using a phantom, TLD or computer software.

E It is a requirement to record dose for patients who are scanned.

Q9.17 CONCERNING CT

A A larger voxel size improves spatial resolution.

B Lower noise levels degrade the image, impairing the ability to visualise small and low contrast detail.

C Image noise is measured using a uniform phantom.

D By increasing the pitch the image unsharpness is reduced.

E By reducing the acquisition slice thickness the noise is increased if the dose is kept constant.

Q9.18 SCATTER WITHIN A CT SCANNER ROOM IS

A Relatively high due to large tissue volumes imaged.

B High because of the high kV used.

C High due to the long scan times.

D Lowest close to the gantry aperture.

E Reduced at the end of the bed due to absorption of scatter by the patient.

Q9.19 CONCERNING RADIATION PROTECTION IN A CT SCANNING ROOM

A Any individual in the room during scanning must wear an apron of 0.25 mm Pb equivalent.

B The use of a thyroid collar has little effect on radiation protection.

C Extremity monitors can be used to measure dose to fingers close to the scan plane.

D The use of the lowest exposure factors reduces the dose received by the patient and the operator.

E Lead glasses are advocated when close to the scan plane.

Q9.20 REGARDING QUALITY ASSURANCE ON CT SCANNERS

A CT number calibration is required to ensure that the CT numbers in the image are correctly calibrated in Hounsfield units (HU).

B CT number calibration is performed using a star resolution grid.

C The focal spot size can be measured using a QC phantom.

D Spatial resolution can be tested by scanning special test objects within the phantom.

E The CT dose index can be measured using a 10 cm pencil ionisation chamber.

Answers

A9.1 THE FOLLOWING FACTORS AFFECT THE SPATIAL RESOLUTION OF CT

A True.

B True – The narrower the slice the narrower the structure which can be resolved.

C True – The smaller the pixel, the smaller the structure which can be resolved.

D False – Windowing improves contrast of specific tissues of interest.

E True.

A9.2 CONCERNING SPATIAL RESOLUTION OF THE CT SCANNER

A True – The greater the noise the less the spatial resolution.

B False – If two structures occupying one voxel are of differing densities their densities will be averaged out, therefore reducing resolution.

C True.

D True.

E False – Patient movement during scanning can affect spatial resolution.

A9.3 THE FOLLOWING ARE TRUE OF CONTRAST IN CT IMAGING

A True.

B False – Air is a negative contrast agent.

C False – They are positive contrast agents.

D True.

E True – Reducing slice thickness increases noise.

A9.4 CONCERNING CT SCANNER COMPONENTS

A False – Tube loading is considerably higher.

B True – The beam is collimated into a fan beam.

C True – This configuration negates the anode heel effect.

D False – The collimators are motorised so slice width can be varied.

E True.

A9.5 THE FOLLOWING FACTORS ARE MEASURED DURING A CT SCAN

A True.

B True.

C True.

D False.

E False.

A9.6 THE FOLLOWING FACTORS ARE USED TO CALCULATE DOSE LENGTH PRODUCT IN CT

A True.

B True.

C True.

D False.

E True – Different regions of the body have different CTDI.

A9.7 THE FOLLOWING CT MEASUREMENTS MATCH THEIR UNITS

A False – CT dose index is measured in mGy.

B False – DLP is measured in mGy.cm.

C True.

D True.

E True.

KEY CONCEPT

CT DOSE MEASUREMENT

Dose parameters used in CT are CT dose index (CTDI) and dose length product (DLP). CTDI is allocated per slice during measurements with a phantom. From this dose length product can be calculated using slice thickness, number of slices and the mAs. Calculations from these values can be used to estimate the effective dose.

A9.8 CONCERNING THE VOXEL IN CT IMAGING

A True.

B True.

C False – Monitors can only display in two dimensions although graphics software can make images appear in 3D.

D True.

E True.

A9.9 THE FOLLOWING METHODS CAN BE USED FOR IMAGE PRODUCTION IN CT

A True.

B False – This is used in digital subtraction angiography with image intensifiers.

C True.

D True.

E False – Pulse height analysers are used in gamma cameras.

A9.10 REGARDING CT IMAGE ARTEFACTS

A False – Stationary high attenuation objects give rise to star artefacts.

B True – Moving objects give rise to streak artefacts.

C True.

D True.

E False – It will produce a streak artefact.

A9.11 THE FOLLOWING ARE CAUSES OF ARTEFACT IN CT SCAN IMAGES

A True.

B True.

C True.

D False.

E True.

A9.12 THE FOLLOWING ARE TRUE OF DETECTORS USED IN CT

A False.

B False – Sodium iodide detectors have now been largely replaced with other scintillation crystals that have better efficiency and less afterglow.

KEY CONCEPT

CT ARTEFACTS AND THEIR CAUSES

- **Star artefacts** are caused by stationary high attenuating objects such as metal.
- **Streak artefacts** are caused by any motion whether it be organ, patient or abnormal unaccounted scanner movement.
- **Partial voluming** is caused by two differently attenuating structures occupying one voxel. This results in the measured attenuation being an average of the two.
- **Ring artefacts** are caused by faulty detectors. The malfunctioning detector will falsely produce a ring in an image as it rotates 360 degrees.
- **Beam hardening** results in the centre of an image having lower CT numbers due to the beam having been attenuated as it passes through the cross section. Special computer programs reduce this to an extent before the image is displayed.
- **Geometrical artefacts** are caused by the diverging CT slices being wider at the edges or narrower at the centre. This means slices may either overlap at the edge or have a gap between them at the centre. This results in either overlapping or absent information.
- **Aliasing artefacts** are due to very sharp and high contrast structure boundaries being displayed as a lower contrast series of lines or streaks.

C True.

D True.

E False – They operate at high atmospheric pressures.

A9.13 THE FOLLOWING ARE TRUE OF DOSE IN CT IMAGING

A False – Reducing slice thickness requires increased mAs to provide enough photons to produce a useful image.

B True – To reduce noise either the mAs or scan time needs to be increased thus increasing patient dose.

C True – Due to the increased patient attenuation the mAs or scan time needs to be increased.

D True.

E True – The slice width is reduced to increase the resolution.

A9.14 REGARDING CT DOSIMETRY

A   False – It is the integral of the dose along the axis of the patient from a single slice *divided* by the nominal thickness of the slice.

B   True.

C   False – $CTDI_W$ is measured in mGy.

D   True.

E   False – The organ dose can be estimated by multiplying the CTDI by the appropriate conversion factors.

A9.15 CONCERNING CT DOSES, THE FOLLOWING ARE TRUE

A   True – Doubling the tube current would double the dose.

B   True – As the gantry rotation time increases the CT dose increases.

C   False – CT dose is inversely proportional to the pitch.

D   True.

E   False – As the kVp increases the CT dose increases.

A9.16 REGARDING CT:

A   False – Under IR(ME)R the DRLs for all examinations are required.

B   True.

C   False – For similar image quality multi-slice scanners are slightly higher dose than single slice scanners.

D   True.

E   True – Most CT scanners display DLP or CTDI.

A9.17 CONCERNING CT

A   False – A smaller voxel size improves spatial resolution.

B   False – Higher noise levels impair the ability to visualise low contrast detail.

C   True.

D   False – Increasing the pitch causes greater unsharpness.

E   True – If the slice thickness is reduced the dose needs to be increased to keep the noise level constant.

A9.18 SCATTER WITHIN A CT SCANNER ROOM IS

A True.

B True.

C True.

D False – The highest scatter is produced close to the gantry aperture.

E True.

A9.19 CONCERNING RADIATION PROTECTION IN A CT SCANNING ROOM

A False – An apron of 0.35 mm Pb is required.

B False – A thyroid collar should be worn.

C True.

D True.

E True.

A9.20 REGARDING QUALITY ASSURANCE ON CT SCANNERS

A True – This is performed by scanning a phantom containing a number of objects of known composition and density and measuring the mean CT value within each object in the image.

B False – This is performed using a QC phantom.

C False – The focal spot size measurement can be made with a stationary tube and a pinhole or a star resolution grid.

D True – A tissue or water equivalent phantom containing either an edge, bead, wire or resolution bar is used.

E True – CTDI is a quantity which is a measure of total dose from a single slice.

CHAPTER 10
Mammography

Q10.1 THE FOLLOWING ARE TRUE OF MAMMOGRAPHIC EQUIPMENT

A The focal spot size is fixed.

B The size of the air gap can be altered.

C The maximum compression permissible of the breast is 200 Newtons (N).

D Grids are not used in mammography.

E The x-ray tube is made from glass.

Q10.2 REGARDING THE FILM–SCREEN COMBINATIONS USED IN MAMMOGRAPHY

A Double emulsion film is used to improve resolution.

B A single screen is used.

C A vacuum is applied to ensure good film/grid contact.

D Films with high gamma are used.

E Films with wide exposure latitude are used to detect as much pathology as possible.

Q10.3 REGARDING COMPRESSION IN MAMMOGRAPHY

A Compression is mandatory in all patients having mammography.

B Compression reduces object–film distance.

C Compression results in good immobilisation of the breast.

D Compression is necessary as mammography is a relatively short exposure.

E Compression increases geometrical unsharpness.

Q10.4 CONCERNING MAMMOGRAPHY

A The dose is so low there is no increased risk of breast cancer.

B The mean dose to the average breast should be less than 2.5 mGy per exposure.

C K edge filters are used.

D The glandular breast tissue is relatively resistant to radiation damage.

E A molybdenum filter cannot be used when a molybdenum target is used.

Q10.5 CONCERNING MAMMOGRAPHY

A The anode heel effect is detrimental.

B An automated exposure control is utilised in mammography.

C A molybdenum target with a molybdenum filter is typically used to image large breasts.

D   Typical resolution in film/screen mammography is between 15 to 20 line pairs/mm.

E   A tungsten target with a rhodium filter is used to image small breasts.

Q10.6 CONCERNING MAMMOGRAPHIC FILM DEVELOPMENT

A   Increasing the developer temperature decreases film fog.

B   Increasing the cycle time increases film contrast to a certain point.

C   Increasing the cycle time decreases film contrast after a certain point.

D   Increasing the developer temperature or concentration reduces film speed.

E   It can be undertaken in a general radiography processing machine.

Q10.7 CONCERNING RADIATION DOSE IN MAMMOGRAPHY

A   The radiation dose is quoted in terms of the effective dose.

B   The radiation dose is measured in mGy.

C   The national dose reference level in the UK is 5 mGy.

D   The dose must be < 2.5 mGy per film for a standard breast in the UK NHS breast screening programme.

E   The glandular tissue in the breast is the most sensitive to radiation.

Q10.8 WEEKLY QUALITY ASSURANCE TESTS PERFORMED IN MAMMOGRAPHY INCLUDE

A Image quality.

B Stereotactic localising device.

C Automatic exposure control with thickness variation.

D Film/screen contact.

E Cassette sensitivity and artefacts.

Q10.9 DAILY QUALITY CONTROL CHECKS IN MAMMOGRAPHY INCLUDE

A Cassette cleaning.

B Compression force.

C Small field digital tests.

D Densitometer calibration.

E Film processor sensitometry.

Q10.10 COMMON FILM ARTEFACTS IN MAMMOGRAPHY INCLUDE

A Film fog.

B Finger marks.

C Dust on the screens.

D Processor roller marks.

E Dust on the filter.

Answers

A10.1 THE FOLLOWING ARE TRUE OF MAMMOGRAPHIC EQUIPMENT

A   False – The focal spot size is variable. Routinely 0.3 mm is used or 0.1 mm when magnifying regions of interest.

B   True – To magnify regions of interest a larger air gap is used.

C   True.

D   False – Grids are used in mammography.

E   True.

A10.2 REGARDING THE FILM–SCREEN COMBINATIONS USED IN MAMMOGRAPHY

A   False – A single emulsion film is used.

B   True.

C   False – A vacuum is applied to the cassette; however, it is to ensure good film/screen contact.

D   True.

E   False – Narrow latitude film is used.

KEY CONCEPT

FILM GAMMA

Film gamma is inversely related to film latitude.

A10.3 REGARDING COMPRESSION IN MAMMOGRAPHY

A   False – In very rare situations such as skin ulceration or surgical wounds compression is not undertaken at the expense of image quality.

B   True.

C   True.

D   False – Mammographic exposures are relatively long.

E   False – Compression reduces geometrical unsharpness.

KEY CONCEPT
K-EDGE FILTERS

K-edge filters are effectively 'blind' to the characteristic radiation produced by targets of the same material. Therefore transmission of desired photon energies can occur while good filtration of other energies can still be obtained.

A10.4 CONCERNING MAMMOGRAPHY

A   False – There is an increased risk of inducing breast cancer.

B   True – The mean dose to each average breast is around 2.0 mGy per mammogram.

C   True.

D   False – Glandular breast tissue is highly sensitive and at risk of radiation damage.

E   False.

A10.5 CONCERNING MAMMOGRAPHY

A   False – The anode heel effect is useful as the target is aligned so that the more intense component of the beam is aimed at the thicker part of the breast.

B   True.

C   False.

D   True.

E   False – This combination is suitable for larger breasts.

A10.6 CONCERNING MAMMOGRAPHIC FILM DEVELOPMENT

A   False – Fog will increase.

B   True – Film contrast will increase to a certain point then decrease.

C   True – As above.

D   False – Speed increases.

E   False.

KEY CONCEPT

X-RAY SPECTRA FOR OPTIMUM IMAGING

Anode	Anode K-edges (keV)	Filter	Beam energy	Breast size/thickness
Molybdenum	α17.4 β20.0	Molybdenum	Lowest	Smallest
Molybdenum	α17.4 β20.0	Rhodium	↓	↓
Rhodium	α20.2 β23.2	Rhodium		
Tungsten	α59.3 β67.2	Rhodium	Highest	Largest

A10.7 CONCERNING RADIATION DOSE IN MAMMOGRAPHY

A False – Radiation dose in mammography is the mean glandular dose (MGD).

B True.

C False – The DRL for mammography is 3.5 mGy.

D True.

E True.

KEY CONCEPT

RADIATION DOSE IN MAMMOGRAPHY

Mean glandular dose (MGD)
Glandular tissue within the breast tissue is most sensitive to radiation. Therefore, the risk from mammography is indicated by the mean adsorbed dose to the glandular tissue within the breast. This is measured in milligray (mGy).

The DRL for mammography in the UK is 3.5 mGy. This is the average dose for a lateral oblique view on a female with 55 mm compressed breast thickness.

A10.8 WEEKLY QUALITY ASSURANCE TESTS PERFORMED IN MAMMOGRAPHY INCLUDE

A   True.

B   True.

C   True.

D   False – This is checked every 6–12 months.

E   False – This is checked every 6–12 months.

A10.9 DAILY QUALITY CONTROL CHECKS IN MAMMOGRAPHY INCLUDE

A   True.

B   False – This is included in the physics system checks which occur monthly.

KEY CONCEPT

MAMMOGRAPHY QUALITY CONTROL

Daily checks
- AEC.
- Film processor densitometry.
- Small field digital tests.
- Cassette cleaning.
- Inspection of breast support table and associated equipment.

Weekly checks
- Image quality.
- Stereotactic localising device.
- AEC consistency with thickness variation.

Monthly tests
- Mechanical safety and function of the compressive device.
- Densitometer calibration.

Every 6–12 months
- Cassette sensitivity and artefacts.
- Film/screen contact.
- Film illuminator output.
- Darkroom safe handling time.
- Darkroom light leakage.

C True.

D False – This is checked monthly.

E True.

A10.10 COMMON FILM ARTEFACTS IN MAMMOGRAPHY INCLUDE

A False.

B False.

C True.

D True.

E True.

CHAPTER 11

Fluoroscopy

Q11.1 THE FOLLOWING ARE TRUE OF IMAGE INTENSIFIERS

A   Light photons are accelerated from the negative input to the positive output screen.

B   Incident x-rays are directly converted into electrons.

C   Each x-ray photon is converted into a single light photon.

D   The image intensifier contains xenon gas to ensure good electron beam focusing.

E   The output screen is coated with a phosphor screen similar in size to the input phosphor.

Q11.2 CONCERNING IMAGE INTENSIFIERS

A Electrons are emitted from the photocathode.

B The input phosphor is made from caesium iodide.

C The output phosphor is made from zinc cadmium sulphide.

D The potential difference is approximately 25 kV.

E The output phosphor is coated with a thin metal layer to prevent back-scatter of light from the output phosphor reaching the input phosphor.

Q11.3 THE FOLLOWING ARE TRUE OF THE ELECTRON BEAM IN THE IMAGE INTENSIFIER

A The electron beam is focused down in size onto the output phosphor by a series of optical mirrors.

B The electron beam is formed when light photons displace electrons from the negatively charged photocathode.

C The electrons travel at a constant speed.

D The electron intensity striking the output phosphor is uniform.

E The electron beam cannot be affected by external magnetic or electrical fields.

Q11.4 REGARDING THE BRIGHTNESS GAIN OF THE IMAGE INTENSIFIER

A Increasing the kVp between the input and output screen will increase the brightness gain.

B Increasing the exposure rate will increase the brightness gain.

C It is defined as the brightness of the output phosphor divided by the input phosphor.

D Can be increased by reducing the output phosphor size in relation to the input phosphor.

E It is affected by the flux gain.

Q11.5 THE FOLLOWING ARE TRUE OF IMAGE MAGNIFICATION

A The brightness will be constant if the exposure factors are kept constant when magnifying an image.

B Magnification can be modified by altering the potential across the intermediate focusing electrodes.

C Skin dose increases with image magnification.

D The size of the output phosphor is altered during magnification.

E The electron beam cross-over point is fixed.

Q11.6 THE FOLLOWING ARE TRUE OF 'VIGNETTING'

A It results in the centre of an image being less bright than the edges.

B Is caused by loss of the electrons in the periphery of the electron beam.

C Is caused by loss of light from the periphery during focusing.

D It can be reduced by curving the input phosphor screen.

E It is reduced by strict quality control.

Q11.7 THE FOLLOWING ARE TRUE OF THE IMAGE INTENSIFIER

A   A small vacuum filled gap is situated between the input phosphor and photocathode.

B   The image produced on the input phosphor is inverted by the time it reaches the output phosphor.

C   The modern intensifier gives a brightness gain of around 100.

D   The conversion factor is the brightness of the output phosphor divided by the flux gain.

E   Minification gain is the area of the output phosphor screen divided by the area of the input phosphor screen.

Q11.8 CONCERNING QUALITY CONTROL OF THE IMAGE INTENSIFIER

A   Resolution can be measured using a line pair test object.

B   Resolution in an image is better at the edges compared to the centre.

C   Resolution can be measured via the modulation transfer function.

D   The modulation transfer function can only be calculated for an entire system and not its constituent parts/stages.

E   Lag causes blurring of moving parts within the image.

Q11.9 THE FOLLOWING STATEMENTS ARE TRUE REGARDING PATIENT DOSE AND THE IMAGE INTENSIFIER

A   The automatic brightness control can increase patient dose.

B   Filters are not used in image intensification equipment.

C   Pulsed fluoroscopy reduces patient dose.

D Typical skin dose rate for an average sized patient is 5 to 15 mGy/ minute.

E Collimation will not alter the surface entrance dose rate; however, it will reduce the effective dose.

Q11.10 REGARDING FLAT PLATE DIGITAL FLUOROSCOPY

A X-ray photons are not converted to light photons at any stage.

B The input phosphor is commonly caesium iodide.

C Amorphous silicon panels convert light photons into electrons.

D There is little or no geometric distortion compared to conventional image intensifiers.

E The dynamic range can be up to 10 times better than conventional image intensifiers.

Q11.11 THE FOLLOWING ARE TRUE OF FLAT PLATE DIGITAL FLUOROSCOPY

A A round image is produced.

B The dynamic range is better than conventional image intensifiers.

C Flat plate systems require increased patient dose compared to conventional image intensifiers.

D Variation of field size alters image noise.

E Collimation does not alter effective dose.

Answers

A11.1 THE FOLLOWING ARE TRUE OF IMAGE INTENSIFIERS

A False – Electrons are accelerated from the negative input screen to the positive output screen.

B False – Incident x-rays are first converted into light photons.

C False – Each absorbed x-ray photon is converted into approximately 400 light photons.

D False – Within the image intensifier tube is a vacuum.

E False – The output phosphor is around one-tenth the size of the input phosphor. This is part of the intensification process in that the accelerated electrons are focused down onto a smaller screen, resulting in a brighter image.

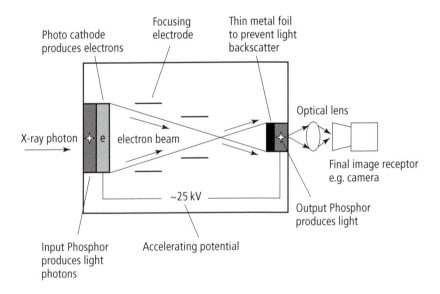

FIGURE 11.1 A schematic view of the image intensifier

A11.2 CONCERNING IMAGE INTENSIFIERS

A True.

B True.

C True.

D True.

E True – This would reduce image quality if light produced in the output phosphor were to scatter back and reach the input phosphor.

A11.3 THE FOLLOWING ARE TRUE OF THE ELECTRON BEAM IN THE IMAGE INTENSIFIER

A False – The electron beam is indeed focused down in size onto the output phosphor. This is achieved by a series of negatively charged circumferentially reducing electrodes.

B True.

C False – The electrons are accelerated towards the output phosphor.

D False – The centre of the electron beam is more intense than the periphery as some peripheral electrons are lost during the electron focusing process. This process is called 'vignetting'.

E False.

A11.4 REGARDING THE BRIGHTNESS GAIN OF THE IMAGE INTENSIFIER

A True.

B False.

C True.

D True – However, the image will be of reduced quality. This is called the minification gain.

E True – Flux gain is due to the increased amount of light photons produced by accelerating the electrons.

A11.5 THE FOLLOWING ARE TRUE OF IMAGE MAGNIFICATION

A False – The brightness of the magnified image will reduce.

B True.

C True.

D False – The size of the output phosphor is fixed.

E False – The electron beam cross-over point can be altered to magnify the image.

A11.6 THE FOLLOWING ARE TRUE OF 'VIGNETTING'

A False.

B True.

C True – The image from the output phosphor is focused through a series of lenses onto image capturing devices such as cameras or x-ray film.

D True – This helps tightly focus the emerging electron beam.

E True – Misaligned focusing electrodes and external electromagnetic forces can cause the electron beam to stray.

A11.7 THE FOLLOWING ARE TRUE OF THE IMAGE INTENSIFIER

A False – The photocathode directly opposes the input phosphor to reduce light divergence and hence image degradation.

B True – The electron beam converges, crosses over then diverges.

C False – The modern intensifiers deliver a brightness gain greater than 10 000.

D False – The conversion factor is the brightness of the output phosphor divided by the input dose rate.

E False – Minification gain is the area of the input phosphor screen divided by the area of the output phosphor screen.

A11.8 CONCERNING QUALITY CONTROL OF THE IMAGE INTENSIFIER

A True.

B False.

C True.

D False – The MTF can be calculated for each stage.

E True.

A11.9 THE FOLLOWING STATEMENTS ARE TRUE REGARDING PATIENT DOSE AND THE IMAGE INTENSIFIER

A True.

B False – Filters such as aluminium or copper are used to reduce patient dose.

C True.

D True.

E True – The entrance dose rate will not reduce but the effective dose will decrease as the irradiated surface area is smaller.

A11.10 REGARDING FLAT PLATE DIGITAL FLUOROSCOPY

A False – X-ray photons are converted into light by the input phosphor.

B True.

C True.

D True – As it is a flat plate there is little or no opportunity for geometrical distortion.

E True.

A11.11 THE FOLLOWING ARE TRUE OF FLAT PLATE DIGITAL FLUOROSCOPY

A False – The plate is rectangular so the image will be rectangular.

B True.

C False.

D False – Varying field size does not alter image noise.

E False.

CHAPTER 12

Radionuclide imaging

Q12.1 THE FOLLOWING STATEMENTS ARE TRUE OF THE RADIONUCLIDE TECHNETIUM-99M

A   It is produced in a cyclotron.

B   It can easily be attached to physiological molecules.

C   It has a half-life of eight hours.

D   It emits gamma rays principally at 140 keV.

E   As well as gamma emission a beta particle is also emitted when it decays to technetium-99.

Q12.2 THE FOLLOWING ARE TRUE OF POSITRON EMITTERS

A   They are produced in a nuclear reactor.

B   Upon decay they emit positive beta particles.

C   They are used in positron emission tomography (PET).

D   Their nuclei are proton deficient.

E   They directly emit two gamma photons of 511 keV.

Q12.3 THE FOLLOWING ENTITIES ARE COMMONLY USED FOR NUCLEAR MEDICINE IMAGING

A Alpha particles.

B Negative beta particles.

C Positive beta particles.

D Gamma photons.

E X-ray photons.

Q12.4 THE FOLLOWING ARE TRUE OF KRYPTON-81M

A It is a liquid at normal atmospheric pressure and room temperature.

B It has a half-life of 13 seconds.

C It is a daughter product of Rubidium-81.

D It emits gamma photons at 190 keV.

E It is produced in a generator adjacent to the patient.

Q12.5 THE FOLLOWING ARE DESIRABLE PROPERTIES OF RADIOPHARMACEUTICALS

A Pure gamma emission.

B Very high energy emission.

C A long half-life.

D For solid organ imaging there should be increased or reduced uptake in pathological tissue compared to normal tissue.

E Single energy of gamma emission.

Q12.6 CONCERNING THE BIOLOGICAL HALF-LIFE (T½) OF A RADIONUCLIDE

A It is affected by the patient's renal function.

B It is interchangeable with the term physical half-life.

C It is not important in calculating the effective half-life.

D If the biological half-life is reduced, the patient dose will increase.

E It is variable.

Q12.7 THE FOLLOWING ARE TRUE OF THE PHYSICAL HALF-LIFE OF A RADIONUCLIDE

A It can be altered by binding to a hydrocarbon chain.

B It is affected by body temperature.

C If the effective half-life is also known, the biological half-life can be calculated.

D It is affected by renal function.

E It is used to calculate the administered dose.

Q12.8 THE EFFECTIVE HALF-LIFE OF A RADIONUCLIDE

A Can be calculated if the physical and biological half-lives are known.

B Is the same for every patient.

C Is not affected by rate of excretion.

D Is used to calculate the effective dose received by the patient.

E Is dependent on the activity of the parent radionuclide.

Q12.9 REGARDING RADIONUCLIDE GENERATORS

A It is possible for a generator to produce radionuclides both in solution and as a gas.

B While in the generator and in equilibrium the parent and daughter radionuclides decay at the half-life of the parent.

C They never need to be refilled.

D They should be easily transportable.

E They do not need a sterile interior as the radioactivity will kill any bacteria.

Q12.10 REGARDING DOSE RECEIVED IN NUCLEAR MEDICINE

A It is expressed as effective dose.

B It is measured in megabecquerels.

C It is dependent on the radioactivity administered.

D It is dependent on the clearance of the radiopharmaceutical.

E The doses received in nuclear medicine cause negligible risk of malignancy.

Q12.11 THE GAMMA CAMERA SCINTILLATION CRYSTAL

A Is commonly made from sodium iodide.

B Is deliberately rendered impure by adding small amounts of elements such as thallium.

C Exhibits fluorescence when exposed to gamma radiation.

D Emits photons of shorter wavelength than that of the incident gamma photons.

E Is robust and waterproof.

Q12.12 THE FOLLOWING STATEMENTS REGARDING IMAGE QUALITY USING THE GAMMA CAMERA ARE TRUE

A If scattered gamma rays are detected and used in image formation they will reduce image contrast.

B The closer the gamma camera head to the patient the better the resolution.

C Resolution can be increased by using a thicker crystal.

D Sensitivity can be increased by using a thicker crystal.

E Resolution can be tested using a thin linear trough filled with technetium-99m.

Q12.13 THE FOLLOWING ARE TRUE OF THE GAMMA CAMERA

A The purpose of the pulse height analyser is to filter out signal from scattered radiation.

B Different energy gamma rays from different radionuclides can be detected simultaneously.

C The purpose of the collimator is to remove scattered radiation.

D The photomultiplier tube converts light photons into electrical signals.

E Light photons produced in the crystal from a gamma photon only illuminate one photomultiplier tube.

Q12.14 REGARDING QUALITY CONTROL OF THE GAMMA CAMERA

A Uniformity of field is tested using a flood field phantom.

B A faulty photomultiplier tube appears as a linear defect in the image.

C A bar phantom can test both linearity and resolution.

D The intrinsic resolution of a gamma camera is typically 3–4 mm.

E By using collimators in radionuclide imaging spatial resolution is reduced.

Q12.15 REGARDING THE COLLIMATOR USED IN NUCLEAR IMAGING

A The smaller the width of the holes in a collimator the higher the resolution.

B The larger the width of the holes in a collimator the higher the sensitivity.

C   The use of collimators limits spatial resolution to around 10 mm.

D   Collimator resolution reduces with increasing distance from the patient.

E   Collimators can be used to magnify or minify images.

Q12.16 REGARDING A PARALLEL HOLE COLLIMATOR

A   Resolution is increased by lengthening the holes.

B   Resolution is decreased by reducing the diameter of the holes.

C   Its principal role is to absorb scattered radiation.

D   Collimator sensitivity is constant with distance.

E   Collimators define the geometrical field of view of the gamma camera.

Q12.17 REGARDING SINGLE PHOTON EMISSION TOMOGRAPHY (SPECT)

A   A gamma camera is used as the detector.

B   The camera constantly rotates around the patient during image acquisition.

C   Back projection is used in image formation.

D   Planar views are reconstructed to form a 3D image.

E   Contrast is improved compared to single gamma camera images.

Q12.18 REGARDING POSITRON EMISSION TOMOGRAPHY (PET)

A   The PET scanner detects positrons.

B   The purpose of the PET scanner is to detect single emission events.

C   Collimation is similar to that of a gamma camera.

D   Image noise is less than that produced by the gamma camera.

E   PET tracer production needs to be on site or nearby as they have short half-lives.

Q12.19 REGARDING THE DETECTION OF GAMMA PHOTONS

A   To distinguish between photons that have only small differences in energy the detector must have a high energy resolution.

B   For resolution to occur between two photons of differing energy their energies must be sufficiently different to lie outside each other's photopeak spread.

C   A detector with a large dead time is required to measure high count rates.

D   An ionisation chamber can detect gamma photons.

E   A Geiger-Müller tube can be used to detect gamma photons.

Q12.20 THE FOLLOWING ARE TRUE OF SINGLE PHOTON EMISSION COMPUTED TOMOGRAPHY (SPECT)

A   It produces two dimensional images.

B   Noise levels are greater than conventional gamma camera images.

C   Spatial resolution is better than conventional computerised tomography using x-rays.

D   Superimposition of overlying structures is a problem.

E   Image acquisition is performed using rotating detectors.

Q12.21 CONCERNING POSITRON EMISSION TOMOGRAPHY

A   Annihilation photons are detected using a ring of detectors.

B   Annihilation photons have energy of 511 keV.

C   Annihilation photons are directly produced by unstable nuclei.

D   Scintillation detectors are made from bismuth germinate.

E   Can be combined with conventional x-ray computerised tomography equipment.

Q12.22 REGARDING THE MEDICINES (ADMINISTRATION OF RADIOACTIVE SUBSTANCES) REGULATIONS 1978

A   Any fully qualified doctor may administer radioactive medicinal products.

B   A radioactive medicinal product is defined as a medicinal product which contains or generates a radioactive substance.

C   The Administration of Radioactive Substances Advisory Committee (ARSAC) certificate is issued by the employer.

D   An ARSAC licence is valid for six years.

E   An ARSAC research licence is valid for two years.

Q12.23 ARSAC CERTIFICATES

A Specify the purpose for which the radioactive substance can be administered.

B The application for an ARSAC licence must be signed by a Radiation Protection Supervisor.

C The employer is responsible for ensuring that the relevant clinicians hold an ARSAC licence.

D The ARSAC certificate holder is responsible for discharging the radioactive patient with the appropriate advice.

E There are three categories of certificates: for diagnostic procedures, therapeutic procedures or research.

Q12.24 CONCERNING NUCLEAR MEDICINE

A The regulatory authority for the use, storage and disposal of radioactive materials is the Environment Agency in England and Wales.

B Aqueous liquid can be disposed of into the sewer.

C Women of child bearing age receiving treatment should be advised regarding future pregnancy.

D Lead aprons are a necessity, providing radiation protection.

E A child should receive a radiopharmaceutical of less activity.

Q12.25 CONCERNING NUCLEAR MEDICINE

A The absorbed dose is calculated from the physical properties of the radionuclide and the bio-distribution data.

B The physical half-life is the result of physical decay and biological clearance.

C The effective half-life cannot be longer than the physical half-life or the biological half-life.

D Absorbed dose is measured in Sv.

E Effective dose is measured in Gy.

Q12.26 THE EFFECTIVE DOSE IN NUCLEAR MEDICINE

A Is 1–10 Gy for common radionuclide procedures with ^{99m}Tc labelled radiopharmaceuticals.

B Is 3–5 Gy for bone scans.

C Is 1–2 Gy for renal studies.

D Is 3–7 Gy for heart studies.

E Is 5–10 Gy for brain scans.

Q12.27 CONCERNING NUCLEAR MEDICINE

A Diagnostic reference levels are not dose limits.

B DRLs are produced by the Administration of Radioactive Substances Advisory Committee.

C DRLs should not be exceeded except in particular circumstances.

D All doses must be kept As Low As Reasonably Practicable.

E Bladder doses can be minimised by drinking plenty of fluid and frequent bladder emptying.

Q12.28 RADIATION PROTECTION IN NUCLEAR MEDICINE

A   Before an MIBG scan, blocking the thyroid with potassium iodide will reduce the effective dose.

B   The activity administered for a child should be reduced according to age.

C   After administration of radionuclides with a long half-life, women are advised to avoid pregnancy for one year.

D   Breast feeding should be stopped for 24 hours if procedures with high activities of ^{99m}Tc are used.

E   The Ionising Radiation Medical Exposure Regulations 2000 provides for the protection of staff.

Q12.29 WHEN HANDLING AND INJECTING RADIOPHARMACEUTICALS

A   Preparation of radiopharmaceuticals should be carried out behind lead glass or thick perspex.

B   Lead aprons should be worn.

C   A thermoluminescent device is not required for dosimetry.

D   Pot shields and syringe shields should be used.

E   Safe disposal of sharps is required.

Q12.30 FOLLOWING ADMINISTRATION OF RADIOPHARMACEUTICALS

A   Patients become a source of external radiation from beta emitters.

B   There are restrictions on contact with children and pregnant women.

C   Incontinent patients can easily be treated with ^{131}I for thyrotoxicosis as outpatients.

D Urine, sweat, faeces, saliva and blood are often radioactive.

E Advice should be given to reduce the risk of radioactive contamination.

Q12.31 IN RADIONUCLIDE IMAGING, SENSITIVITY IS

A The ability to produce an image where count values are equal in every pixel when irradiated by a uniform source.

B A measure of the sharpness of the image.

C A measure of the spatial distortion of an image.

D A measure of the proportion of gamma rays emitted from a radionuclide source which are detected within the photopeak of the collimated gamma camera.

E The ability of the gamma camera to register the count rate linearly in response to incident count rates.

Q12.32 QUALITY ASSURANCE IN RADIONUCLIDE IMAGING INVOLVES MEASURING

A Uniformity.

B Spatial resolution.

C Linearity.

D Sensitivity.

E Count rate capability.

Answers

A12.1 THE FOLLOWING STATEMENTS ARE TRUE OF THE RADIONUCLIDE TECHNETIUM-99M

A False – It is produced in a generator.

B False – Technetium is difficult to attach to physiological molecules.

C False – Technetium-99m has a half-life of six hours.

D True.

E False – It is a metastable radionuclide and therefore decays by gamma emission only.

A12.2 THE FOLLOWING ARE TRUE OF POSITRON EMITTERS

A False – They are produced in a cyclotron.

B True.

C True.

D False – Their nuclei are neutron deficient.

E False – It is the annihilation with nearby electrons that produce two 511 keV photons.

KEY CONCEPT

TECHNETIUM-99M

- Produced by decay of its parent molybdenum-99.
- It can then be eluted from a generator.
- It is a metastable radionuclide and decays by emitting 140 keV gamma photons.
- Has a half-life of six hours.
- Can be labelled to various physiological molecules for imaging purposes.

A12.3 THE FOLLOWING ENTITIES ARE COMMONLY USED FOR NUCLEAR MEDICINE IMAGING

A False – They cannot escape the body.

B False – Negative beta particles are high speed electrons and have very limited imaging potential as their path length in solid tissue is short.

C True – These are positrons.

D True.

E False – X-rays are not used in nuclear imaging.

A12.4 THE FOLLOWING ARE TRUE OF KRYPTON-81M

A False – It is a gas and can be used in ventilation studies.

B True.

C True.

D True.

E True – The half-life of krypton-81m is so short it needs to be produced in a generator located next to the patient.

A12.5 THE FOLLOWING ARE DESIRABLE PROPERTIES OF RADIOPHARMACEUTICALS

A True.

B False – If the energy of the gamma photons is too high, there will be too little attenuation in the detector.

C False – Half-life should not be too long as this will increase patient dose.

D True.

E True – This allows correct detection of true signal. Any other energies detected can be rejected as scatter.

A12.6 CONCERNING THE BIOLOGICAL HALF-LIFE (T½) OF A RADIONUCLIDE

A True.

B False.

C False – Both the physical and biological half-lives are required to calculate the effective half-life.

D False – The shorter the biological half-life the quicker the radionuclide is being eliminated from the patient.

E True.

> ### KEY CONCEPT
>
> #### EFFECTIVE HALF-LIFE, PHYSICAL HALF-LIFE AND BIOLOGICAL HALF-LIFE
>
> - Physical half-life is the actual half-life of the radionuclide atoms and takes no account of physical, chemical and biological conditions.
> - Biological half-life is due to the rate of elimination of the radionuclide atoms from the patient
> - Effective half-life is calculated from the above two half-lives using the following formula:
>
> 1/effective half-life = 1/physical half-life + 1/biological half-life

A12.7 THE FOLLOWING ARE TRUE OF THE PHYSICAL HALF-LIFE OF A RADIONUCLIDE

A False.

B False.

C True.

D False.

E True.

A12.8 THE EFFECTIVE HALF-LIFE OF A RADIONUCLIDE

A True.

B False.

C False – This affects the biological half-life.

D True.

E False.

A12.9 REGARDING RADIONUCLIDE GENERATORS

A True.

B True – The parent and daughter radionuclides are described as being in transient equilibrium.

C False.

D True.

E False.

A12.10 REGARDING DOSE RECEIVED IN NUCLEAR MEDICINE

A   True.

B   False – Effective dose is measured in sieverts.

C   True.

D   True.

E   False.

A12.11 THE GAMMA CAMERA SCINTILLATION CRYSTAL

A   True.

B   True.

C   True.

D   False – The emitted photons from a fluorescent process have lower energy than the incident photon, therefore the wavelength will be longer.

E   False – The crystals are very fragile and are also susceptible to water damage.

KEY CONCEPT

FLUORESCENCE

- The incident photon imparts energy to an electron in the valence band.
- This more energetic electron can jump to a conduction band if it has sufficient energy.
- The electron loses energy and returns from the conduction band to the valence band.
- This process results in a photon being emitted. Its energy will be the difference between the energy levels of the conduction band and the valence band.

A12.12 THE FOLLOWING STATEMENTS REGARDING IMAGE QUALITY USING THE GAMMA CAMERA ARE TRUE

A True.

B True – The closer the gamma camera head the less opportunity emitted gamma rays have to diverge.

C False – Resolution is increased by using a thinner crystal.

D True – The thicker the crystal the more gamma photons will be captured.

E True.

A12.13 THE FOLLOWING ARE TRUE OF THE GAMMA CAMERA

A True – The pulse height analyser is set to only accept pulses within a certain energy range.

B True.

C False – The pulse height analyser removes scattered radiation. The collimator allows the location of the source within the patient to be defined.

D True.

E False – Numerous adjacent photomultiplier tubes may detect the light photons emitted by one gamma photon interaction.

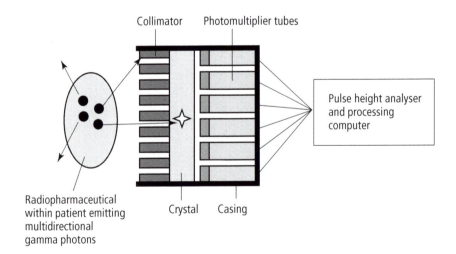

FIGURE 12.1 Schematic view of the gamma camera

A12.14 REGARDING QUALITY CONTROL OF THE GAMMA CAMERA

A True.

B False – It will appear as roughly the shape of the photomultiplier head.

C True.

D True.

E True – Collimators reduce the spatial resolution of the gamma camera from around 3–4 mm to 10 mm.

A12.15 REGARDING THE COLLIMATOR USED IN NUCLEAR IMAGING

A True.

B True.

C True.

D True.

E True – A pinhole collimator can be used to magnify a small area onto the gamma camera head (e.g. thyroid scans). A divergent collimator can image a larger area and project it onto a smaller gamma camera (e.g. lungs).

A12.16 REGARDING A PARALLEL HOLE COLLIMATOR

A True.

B False – The resolution increases by reducing the diameter of the holes.

C False – Its principal role is to allow localisation of the radionuclide within the patient. Scattered radiation is eliminated by energy selection by the pulse height analyser.

D True.

E True.

A12.17 REGARDING SINGLE PHOTON EMISSION TOMOGRAPHY (SPECT)

A True.

B False – It pauses and acquires images in small increments as it rotates around the patient.

C True.

D True.

E True.

A12.18 REGARDING POSITRON EMISSION TOMOGRAPHY (PET)

A False – The PET scanner detects the gamma rays emitted as a result of annihilation events between positrons and electrons.

B False – The concept behind the PET scanner is to simultaneously detect two gamma photons of 511 keV emitted in opposite directions.

C False – Collimation is not required.

D True.

E True – The most commonly used tracer is glucose labelled with fluorine-18 (18-FDG), which has a half-life of only 110 minutes.

A12.19 REGARDING THE DETECTION OF GAMMA PHOTONS

A True.

B True.

C False – A detector with a small dead time is required.

D True.

E True.

A12.20 THE FOLLOWING ARE TRUE OF SINGLE PHOTON EMISSION COMPUTED TOMOGRAPHY (SPECT)

A False – It produces three-dimensional images.

B True – Noise is greater because the images are made up from fewer photons.

C False – It is worse.

D False – In SPECT overlying structures are resolved during 3D reconstruction.

E True – The camera heads rotate around the patient.

A12.21 CONCERNING POSITRON EMISSION TOMOGRAPHY

A True.

B True.

C False – Annihilation photons are produced by positron-electron annihilation events.

D True.

E True – This is PET-CT.

A12.22 REGARDING THE MEDICINES (ADMINISTRATION OF RADIOACTIVE SUBSTANCES) REGULATIONS 1978

A False – Procedures should only be carried out under the supervision of a person holding an ARSAC licence.

B True.

C False – This certificate is issued by the Administration of Radioactive Substances Advisory Committee of the Department of Health.

D False – It is valid for five years.

E True.

A12.23 ARSAC CERTIFICATES

A True – ARSAC certificates are issued to individual clinicians for specified procedures.

B False – The application has to be signed by a Radiation Protection Advisor.

C True.

D True.

E True.

A12.24 CONCERNING NUCLEAR MEDICINE

A True – The Scottish Environment Protection Agency and the Environment and Heritage Service are the responsible regulatory authorities in Scotland and Northern Ireland respectively.

B True.

C True.

D False – Lead aprons are not worn by radiographers in nuclear medicine as they provide little protection.

E True – Administered activity is reduced according to the child's weight.

```
                    KEY CONCEPT
            DISPOSAL OF RADIOACTIVE WASTE
```

Routes of disposal of radioactive waste

This is determined by the Radioactive Substances Act 1993.

- Gas can be disposed of into the atmosphere.
- Aqueous liquid can be disposed of into the sewer.
- Organic liquid must be disposed of via a contractor who has authorisation for the transfer and final disposal of the radioactive substance.
- Solid radioactive waste must be disposed of by a contractor in an incinerator.
- Records of disposal must be sent to the environment agency; these records are available for public viewing.

A12.25 CONCERNING NUCLEAR MEDICINE

A   True – The physical properties of radionuclides are the emissions/energies. The bio-distribution data is the uptake and clearance of the radionuclide which is obtained from temporal sampling.

B   False – Effective half-life is the result of physical decay and biological clearance.

C   True.

D   False – Absorbed dose is measured in Gy.

E   False – Effective dose is measured in Sv.

A12.26 THE EFFECTIVE DOSE IN NUCLEAR MEDICINE

A   False – Effective doses are measured in Sv.

B   False – All these questions are false because of the incorrect units.

C   False.

D   False.

E   False.

A12.27 CONCERNING NUCLEAR MEDICINE

A   True – There are no dose limits for medical exposures, but doses must be kept ALARP for the intended purpose.

B   True.

KEY CONCEPT

DOSIMETRY IN NUCLEAR MEDICINE

- **Absorbed dose** will depend on the cumulated activity in the source organ and the fraction of energy absorbed in the target organ. Measured in **Gy**.
- **Effective doses** are used to consider the different sensitivities of different organs and tissues to stochastic radiation effects. Measured in **Sv**.

The annual average natural background radiation dose in the UK is approximately 2.3 mSv.

Common radionuclide procedures with ^{99m}Tc labelled radiopharmaceuticals are 1–10 mSv. They include the following.
- Renal studies 1–2 mSv.
- Bone scans 3–5 mSv.
- Heart studies 3–7 mSv.
- Brain scans 5–10 mSv.

Some diagnostic procedures involve higher doses as follows.
- Indium imaging 3–20 mSv.
- Thallium imaging 18–37 mSv.

C   True – These include obesity, additional views and SPECT.

D   True.

E   True – This effectively reduces the dose as many radionuclides are excreted by the kidneys.

A12.28 RADIATION PROTECTION IN NUCLEAR MEDICINE

A   True.

B   False – The administered activity should be reduced according to the child's weight

C   False – Women are advised to avoid pregnancy for a few months. The absorbed dose to the foetus should not exceed 1 mGy.

D   True.

E   False – IR(ME)R (2000) provides for the protection of patients. IRR 99 provides for the protection of staff.

A12.29 WHEN HANDLING AND INJECTING RADIOPHARMACEUTICALS

A True.

B False – They provide little protection against high energy gamma radiation.

C False.

D True.

E True.

A12.30 FOLLOWING ADMINISTRATION OF RADIOPHARMACEUTICALS

A False – External radiation is from gamma emitters.

B True – Restricted contact is recommended.

C False – Incontinent patients present a particular problem due to contamination of pads and clothing.

D True.

E True.

A12.31 IN RADIONUCLIDE IMAGING, SENSITIVITY IS

A False – This is uniformity.

B False – This is spatial resolution.

C False – This is spatial linearity.

D True.

E False – This is the count rate capability.

A12.32 QUALITY ASSURANCE IN RADIONUCLIDE IMAGING INVOLVES MEASURING

A True.

B True.

C True.

D True.

E True.

Index

(Q) refers 'questions'; (A) to 'answers', key concepts or definitions.